European Practice in Gynaecology and Obstetrics

Diabetes and pregnancy

In the same series

Invasive carcinoma of the cervix
Volume editor: G. Body
ISBN: 2-84299-306-3

Breech delivery
Volume editor: W. Künzel
ISBN: 2-84299-314-4

Ovulation induction
Volume editor: B. Tarlatzis
ISBN: 2-84299-317-9

Viral infection in pregnancy
Volume editors: G. Donders, B. Stray-Pedersen
ISBN: 2-84299-317-9

Endometrial cancer
Volume editor: P. Bösze
ISBN: 0-444-51361-2

Paediatric and adolescent gynaecology
Volume editor: J.-J. Amy
ISBN: 0-444-51360-4

http://intl.elsevierhealth.com/series/ebcog

European Practice in Gynaecology and Obstetrics

Diabetes and pregnancy

Volume Editor
F.A. Van Assche (Belgium)

L. Aerts (Belgium)
L. Cabero-Roura (Spain)
Ma.J. Cerqueira (Spain)
P. Djerf (Sweden)
U.J. Eriksson (Sweden)
D. Hadden (U.K.)
U. Hanson (Sweden)
K. Holemans (Belgium)

A. Kennedy (U.K.)
C. Lowy (U.K.)
A. Nugent (U.K.)
D.W. Pearson (U.K.)
B. Persson (Sweden)
A. Ross (U.K.)
F.A. Van Assche (Belgium)
J. Verhaeghe (Belgium)

2004

ELSEVIER

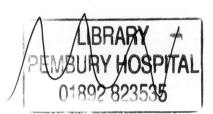

ELSEVIER B.V.
Sara Burgerhartstraat 25
P.O. Box 211, 1000 AE Amsterdam, The Netherlands

First edition 2004

Library of Congress Cataloging in Publication Data
A catalog record form the Library of Congress has been applied for.

British Library Cataloging in Publication Data

W Q 248

Assche, F. A. van
  Diabetes and pregnancy. - (European practice in gynaecology
  and obstetrics ; v. 7)
  1.Diabetes and pregnancy
  I.Title II.European Board and College of Obstetrics and
  Gynaecology
  618.3

  ISBN: 0 444 51513 5

 ∞ The paper used in this publication meets the requirements of ANSI/NISO Z39.48-1992 (Permanence of Paper).
Printed in The Netherlands.

Diabetes and pregnancy

Contributing authors

Volume Editor
F.A. Van Assche (Belgium)

L. Aerts (Belgium)
L. Cabero-Roura (Spain)
Ma.J. Cerqueira (Spain)
P. Djerf (Sweden)
U.J. Eriksson (Sweden)
D. Hadden (U.K.)
U. Hanson (Sweden)
K. Holemans (Belgium)

A. Kennedy (U.K.)
C. Lowy (U.K.)
A. Nugent (U.K.)
D.W. Pearson (U.K.)
B. Persson (Sweden)
A. Ross (U.K.)
F.A. Van Assche (Belgium)
J. Verhaeghe (Belgium)

Scientific committee

J. Lansac (France)
Chairman

J. J. Amy (Belgium), P. Bösze (Hungary), M. Cabero Roura (Spain), W. Dunlop (U.K.),
A. Goverde (Netherlands), I. Milsom (Sweden), F. Nunes (Portugal), K. Schneider (Germany),
B. Tarlatzis (Greece), V. Unzeitig (Czech Republic)

Table of Contents

Preface

Why this collection on "European Practice in Gynaecology and Obstetrics"?

The European Union is evolving nicely.

Under the auspices of the European Board and College of Obstetrics and Gynaecology (EBCOG), recommendations have been published and accepted by the European Union of Medical Specialists (UEMS) in order to standardise the training of gynaecologists and obstetricians in order to ensure quality care and facilitate the exchange amongst physicians in European countries.

It was deemed that a series of books covering obstetrical and gynaecological practice was needed to provide up-to-date information for post-graduate students and the continuing education of specialists.

A common EBCOG and EAGO scientific committee is responsible for the contents of the collection. For each topic, this committee has selected the volume editor and the contributing authors, specialists throughout Europe known for their expertise in their fields. Each chapter is reviewed by external referees to assess the scientific quality of its contents and the evidence-based recommendations.

The authors describe the various types of management used in European practice, as well as the published results. They present those treatments for which a consensus exists; when there is no consensus, they discuss the key elements of the controversy.

In each book, the reader will find a review of the basic science, recent concepts in physiopathology, clinical aspects, treatment and unresolved problems or controversies, as well as the major recent references. A final section provides multiple-choice questions covering each chapter.

We would like our readers to give us their opinions on these books so that we can continue to make this collection a useful tool for students and practising specialists alike.

Professor Jacques Lansac, MD, FRCOG
Chairman of the Scientific Committee

Diabetes and Pregnancy

Prof. Van Assche, MD,Phd,FRCOG,Dr.Hon.c.Athens

Diabetes is increasing in the world and is becoming one of the most important medical diseases in this century, but also the association between diabetes and pregnancy will be more frequent.

Furthermore, an abnormal intra-uterine environment can be responsible for the occurrence in later life. These facts may underline the importance of the EBCOG Elsevier Volume on Diabetes and Pregnancy.

It is important to distinguish pre-existing diabetes and gestational diabetes.

In *pre-existing diabetes* the main management action should be on pre-pregnancy care. A normal diabetic control should be achieved before conception. This perfect diabetic control needs continuity during the whole duration of pregnancy. This can avoid major fetal and maternal complications. It is clear that poor diabetic control before and in the course of pregnancy increases the risk of congenital malformations, but also of an increased perinatal morbidity and mortality.

The fetus is mostly macrosomic, but intra-uterine growth restriction can occur when nefro vascular complications are present. Fetal surveillance by regular obstetrical ultrasound, fetal heart rate monitoring and clinical judgement is an absolute indication.

Diabetes is associated with an increased risk of pre-eclampsia, probably due to an imbalance between tromboxane and prostacyclin and also to the presence of an oxidative stress.

Gestational diabetes is mainly associated with fetal macrosomia, inducing an increased risk for birth trauma.

It is therefore most important to screen for gestational diabetes. This is certainly true for pregnancies at risk, but general screening with the 50 g glucose challenge test is certainly recommended. The final diagnosis of gestational diabetes is made by the oral glucose tolerance test. Treatment should start with diet and addition of insulin therapy is performed when the glycaemia levels are not under control.

The efficient management of diabetes during pregnancy is not only important for the benefit of perinatal outcome, it may also be of benefit for the outcome in later life.

Macrosomia associated with fetal hyper-insulinism may be responsible for a reduced insulin secretion in later life, whereas intra-uterine growth retardation associated with fetal hypo-insulinism may induce insulin resistance in later life; both conditions reflect the fetal origin of adult diseases in the offspring.

Furthermore, gestational diabetes is a risk factor for diabetes in women years after pregnancy.

In conclusion:

Diabetes is a frequent and severe complication during pregnancy. Detection and perfect maternal control, and also constant fetal surveillance are necessary to improve not only perinatal morbidity and mortality, but also maternal morbidity.

Furthermore, control of fetal growth could prevent diseases in adult life in the offspring.

Chapter 1

Gestational diabetes mellitus: pathophysiology, screening and diagnosis, and management

Johan Verhaeghe

Johan Verhaeghe, Department of Obstetrics and Gynaecology, U.Z. Gasthuisberg, Katholieke Universiteit Leuven, 3000 Leuven, Belgium.

Gestational diabetes mellitus: pathophysiology, screening and diagnosis, and management

Johan Verhaeghe*

Abstract.—*Gestational diabetes mellitus (GDM) is any form of diabetes or glucose intolerance with onset or first recognition during pregnancy. The central features of its pathophysiology are: aggravated insulin resistance compared with normal pregnancies, and inadequate insulin secretory response relative to the degree of insulin resistance. GDM is a heterogeneous syndrome, with pathogenetic factors reminiscent of both type 2 and type 1 diabetes. There are several pregestational and gestational clinical risk factors, that include: overweight with central distribution, short stature, age, parity, ethnicity, family history of diabetes, history of PCO syndrome and multiple pregnancy. The prevalence of GDM is dependent on the ethnic composition of the pregnant population and the diagnostic criteria; in the USA, the prevalence is estimated to be 3.5%. Being a frequent and potentially hazardous complication of pregnancy, screening for GDM is recommended. Screening with the glucose challenge test (GCT: 50 g glucose orally, and venous plasma glucose measurement after 60 minutes) between 24 and 28 weeks is superior to risk factor-based screening. Recent modifications of the GCT include: variable cut-off values according to the time since last meal, and the exclusion of "low-risk" women from screening. A fasting plasma glucose measurement between 24 and 28 weeks may be useful as an alternative to the GCT. The diagnosis of GDM is made by an oral glucose tolerance test (OGTT), with either 100 or 75 g of glucose. Using the stricter "Carpenter-Coustan" criteria rather than the original "National Diabetes Data Group" criteria (1979) for the 100-g OGTT, results in a substantial increase of the proportion of pregnant women labeled to have GDM. When using the 75-g OGTT, pregnancy-specific values are recommended rather than the WHO (1980) criteria for nonpregnant subjects. The medical management of GDM consists of prescribing medical nutrition therapy, encouraging moderate exercise and starting glucose monitoring, preferably by self-monitoring of blood glucose (SMBG). Human insulin preparations should be added in case of fasting hyperglycemia, or when SMBG indicates unsatisfactory glycemic control.*

Keywords: gestational diabetes, screening, diagnosis, management, physiopathology.

*Address for correspondence: J. Verhaeghe, Department of Obstetrics and Gynaecology, U.Z. Gasthuisberg, Herestraat 49, Leuven, Belgium. Tel.: +32-16344215, Fax: +32-16344205, E-mail: johan.verhaeghe@uz.kuleuven.ac.be

What is gestational diabetes mellitus (GDM)?

Gestational diabetes mellitus (GDM) is *any form of diabetes mellitus or impaired glucose tolerance (IGT) with first onset or first recognition during the index pregnancy.* Thus, the diagnosis of GDM is independent of the possibility that the diabetes or glucose intolerance may have antedated the pregnancy. Indeed, diabetes or glucose intolerance in women are more frequently discovered during pregnancy than in the nonpregnant state, because of procedures routinely carried out during the antepartum course (history taking, glycosuria testing, plasma glucose testing, glucose challenge and tolerance tests). The definition of GDM is also independent of the severity of the hyperglycemia, and of the possible need of insulin treatment during pregnancy. Finally, it is independent of the possible persistence of hyperglycemia – as diabetes, impaired fasting plasma glucose or impaired glucose tolerance – after delivery. This broad definition of GDM is of great practical value and has boosted research into GDM in obstetric units. The reverse side of this broad definition is that GDM is a heterogeneous syndrome in terms of clinical severity, pathophysiology and pathogenesis (see "Glucose-insulin metabolism in women with GDM: a summary").

Pathophysiology of GDM

■ Maternal glucose-insulin metabolism during normal pregnancy: a summary

Normal pregnancy is characterized by two major alterations in glucose homeostasis. First, there is a continuous transfer of glucose to the conceptus, i.e., the fetus and the placenta. The transplacental glucose transport is facilitated by glucose transporters (GLUTs), mainly GLUT-1 and GLUT-3. Because of the glucose utilization by the conceptus, pregnancy constitutes a state of "accelerated starvation" for the mother: during fasting, glucose levels fall more rapidly than in nonpregnant women while lipolysis and ketogenesis are activated. The second alteration is the development of a state of reduced tissue insulin sensitivity, or "insulin resistance", from the second trimester of pregnancy onward [1]. The insulin resistance during pregnancy comprises both glucose and lipid metabolism. Regarding glucose metabolism, there is resistance to the action of insulin to stimulate glucose utilization by skeletal muscles and adipose tissue, and resistance to the blunting of endogenous glucose production by the liver; these changes occur in lean as well as in obese pregnant women. Regarding lipid metabolism, there is resistance to the action of insulin to inhibit lipolysis and fat oxidation. Tissue insulin resistance results in a gradual and compensatory stimulation of insulin secretion by the pancreatic β-cells: fasting insulin levels, and both first- and second-phase of the insulin response to an intravenous glucose test (IVGTT) are augmented during pregnancy [1]. Insulin clearance accelerates with advancing gestation.

■ Glucose-insulin metabolism in women with GDM: a summary

From a *pathophysiological* point of view, GDM pregnancies are characterized by increased insulin resistance compared with normal pregnancies, as shown by studies using frequently sampled IVGTTs or euglycemic hyperinsulinemic clamps [2]. The insulin resistance affects carbohydrate and lipid metabolism, and presumably protein metabolism as well. In women with GDM, plasma glucose is cleared less effectively by insulin-sensitive tissues, whereas endogenous glucose production by the liver is increased, under basal conditions and during hyperinsulinemia [2]. Fasting plasma FFA levels are raised, and are less dampened by hyperinsulinemia [2]. The insulin resistance was shown to be more dramatic in women with both GDM and chronic hypertension (i.e., hypertension prior to 20 weeks of pregnancy) than in women with GDM alone [3]. Second, while fasting insulin levels are normal or increased in women with GDM, the insulin secretory response to glucose or a meal is inadequate relative to the degree of insulin resistance: in particular, the first-phase insulin response to an oral glucose tolerance test (OGTT) or an IVGTT is deficient compared with normal pregnancies [2]. The impaired insulin secretory response is most evident in lean women with GDM. In contrast, the second-phase insulin response is not reduced in women with GDM compared with weight-matched controls, and was actually found to be increased in some studies. GDM is also characterized by increased concentrations of proinsulin, further demonstrating β-cell functional impairment.

From a *pathogenetic* point of view, the exaggerated insulin resistance could to some extent be explained by overweight/obesity, which is more frequent in women with GDM ("Risk factors for GDM"). Gene mutations that are responsible for MODY (maturity-onset diabetes of the young) – a genetically and clinically heterogeneous group of autosomally dominant, early-onset type 2 diabetes with insulin secretion defects – have also been found in some women with GDM, including glucokinase gene mutations which result in "MODY 2". Glucosinase mutations are believed to account for 3-6% of cases of GDM, and to affect birth weight per se. Other "postreceptor" abnormalities (i.e., defects that occur beyond the binding of insulin to its receptor) have been characterized in some women with GDM. Thus, abnormal tyrosine kinase activity in skeletal muscle has been reported, and a depletion of GLUT-4 (the insulin-responsive glucose transporter) content has been observed in adipocytes of about 50% of women with GDM. On the other hand, auto-antibodies against insulin, islet cells, glutamic acid decarboxylase (GAD_{65}) and/or tyrosine phosphatase (IA2) have been detected in up to 10% of GDM pregnancies, and islet cell-surface antibodies were detected in 31% of GDM patients in another study [4]. More importantly, the presence of auto-antibodies (multiple antibodies, in particular) identified a subgroup of GDM at high risk for subsequent development of type 1 diabetes, as shown in a study from Germany [5]. Thus, pathogenic factors related to both type 2 and type 1 diabetes have been characterized in women with GDM. It appears, therefore, that GDM is pathogenetically a heterogeneous syndrome.

Screening and diagnosis of GDM

■ Screening of GDM

Risk factors for GDM

There are pregestational as well as gestational risk factors for GDM. In the Nurses' Health Study Cohort in the USA [6], comprising 14,613 women, a number of *pregestational* factors were identified that were associated with increased prevalence of GDM: overweight and obesity, weight gain since 18 years of age, increasing age, ethnicity, a family history of diabetes, and current smoking. Factors that conferred at least a doubling of the relative risk were: overweight (BMI 25-29.9 kg/m^2) and obesity (≥ 30), compared with lean women (BMI <20); weight gain of ≥ 10 kg from age 18 years compared with weight gain/loss <5 kg; age ≥ 40 years, compared with 25-29 years; and Asian ethnicity versus Caucasian. The effect of bodyweight appears to interact with ethnicity: overweight was shown to have a larger effect on GDM prevalence in North American Native women than in non-Native women. However, the effect of weight was also demonstrable in a Scandinavian population with a low prevalence of obesity [7]. Excess adipose tissue in GDM women is primarily in the abdominal region ("android" obesity), as shown by an increased waist/hip ratio [8]. In addition to the abovementioned pregestational factors, parity was found to be an independent predictor of GDM in some cohorts [9, 10]. Short stature has been indentified as a risk factor for the development of GDM in several cohorts [7, 11]. Finally, polycystic ovary (PCO) syndrome [12] and chronic hypertension [3] are associated with increased prevalence of GDM. Presumably, many of the pregestational risk factors of GDM are mediated by insulin resistance: overweight/obesity with central distribution, short stature, ethnicity, PCO syndrome, and chronic hypertension. Thus, GDM could be considered as a clinical manifestation of the insulin resistance syndrome, as it shares many of its metabolic components.

Some *pregnancy-associated* characteristics increase the risk of GDM. The most important risk factor is multiple pregnancy: the risk of GDM is about two-fold increased in twin pregnancies versus singleton pregnancies, and appears to be further increased in triplet pregnancies [13]. There is also an association between GDM and hypertensive diseases of pregnancy. In a prospective series of about 3700 healthy nulliparous women, the relative risk of developing hypertensive diseases of pregnancy (gestational hypertension and pre-eclampsia) was 1.54 [95% confidence intervals (CI), 1.28-2.11] in women with GDM compared with non-GDM women [14]. Treatment with β-adrenergic agents and/or corticosteroids for preterm labor increases the risk of meeting the diagnostic criteria for GDM [15]; women on chronic steroid therapy also have a higher risk [16].

Risk factors, obtained by the medical history and the clinical examination, have long been used as a screening method for GDM: if one or more risk factors were abnormal, the patient was referred for a diagnostic test, i.e., an OGTT (see "The diagnosis of GDM"). A recent randomized study demonstrated that universal screening with the glucose challenge test (see "The glucose challenge test (GCT)") was superior to risk factor-based screening: the detection rate of GDM was higher, gestational age at diagnosis was earlier, and overall perinatal oucome was better [17]. The drawback of risk factor-based screening for GDM is that it is dependent on accurate history taking, as well as on the predefined "abnormality" threshold of any predefined clinical risk factor (bodyweight, fetal macrosomia, polyhydramnios, etc.).

The prevalence of GDM

GDM is a frequent complication of pregnancy. The prevalence of GDM in any obstetric unit, region or country depends on the ethnic composition of its population, and, naturally, on the cut-off values used in the diagnostic test (see "The diagnosis of GDM"). Using standard criteria, the prevalence of GDM in the USA in 1988 was calculated to be 3.5% (95% confidence intervals: 2.9-4.0) [18]. In North America, the prevalence of GDM is significantly higher in units/areas that serve pregnant populations with a Latino (Hispanic) and/or Native background. In North America, the UK and Australia, GDM has also been reported to be markedly more prevalent in women with an Asian (Indian subcontinent, Chinese, South-East-Asian) background [6, 9, 10]. Other populations at higher risk include Maori of New Zealand and other Pacific Islanders. The prevalence of GDM in populations from African descent was also found to be higher than that of Caucasians in some [6, 9], but not all [10], studies. In other countries, the prevalence of GDM is somewhat lower than in North America, e.g., 2.0% in an ethnically homogeneous cohort from Korea [11].

Given a prevalence of 2-3.5% or more, GDM is one of the most frequent complications of pregnancy, together with hypertensive diseases (10% or more), premature labor (about 7%) and intra-uterine growth retardation.

The glucose challenge test (GCT)

The GCT was described by O'Sullivan et al, in 1973: 752 pregnant women ingested 50 g of glucose, and had a whole-blood glucose measurement after one hour; they subsequently underwent a diagnostic 100-g OGTT (see "The diagnosis GDM"). A cut-off value of 130 mg/dl after the GCT was defined as the best threshold value, which had a sensitivity of 79% and a specificity of 88% for the subsequent diagnosis of GDM.

Before 1997, the American Diabetes Association (ADA) recommended that all pregnant women should have a GCT. The GCT should be performed between 24 and 28 weeks of pregnancy, in either fasting or nonfasting conditions. Since most laboratories have switched from blood to plasma glucose measurements, a specific plasma glucose cut-off value is needed. A blood glucose value of 130 mg/dl has been converted to a plasma value of 143 mg/dl; using this cut-off value, the GCT was found to have a sensitivity of 83% and a specificity of 87% for the diagnosis of GDM [19], confirming the data of O'Sullivan et al. For simplicity, the ADA recommends using 140 mg/dl (7.8 mmol/l) in a venous plasma sample as the cut-off value. In a study on 704 women, this cut-off value again had a sensitivity of 83% and a specificity of 74% [20]; 17-18% of screened women will have a positive test [10, 21]. To increase the sensitivity of the GCT to about 90%, 130 mg/dl (7.2 mmol/l) has been proposed as the alternative cut-off value; using this cut-off value, 20-25% of screenees will have a positive test [22].

In the latest Clinical Practice Recommendations [23], the ADA recommends a GCT in (1) all women from the age of 25 years, and (2) in women <25 years at "high risk", i.e., women who have an increased weight (the threshold is not defined), or belong to an ethnic group with increased prevalence of GDM (non-Caucasians?), or have a first-degree relative with diabetes, or have a history of glucose intolerance, or a history of poor obstetric outcome (not further defined). Some studies have criticized these recommendations. First, the nonscreened population is a relatively small group (about 10% of the pregnant population in some centers) [24]. Second, the incidence of GDM in the presumed "low-risk" population is not negligible: in one Australian cohort of 573 women, it was found to be 2.8% [25]; in another study on 509 teenage pregnancies, the incidence was

1.2% [26]. Third, the insulin requirement and pregnancy outcome figures in women with a GDM diagnosis were comparable in the "low-risk" category versus the other group [25]. Finally, it adds complexity to the screening procedure.

Naylor et al [10] proposed a screening schema for GDM on the basis of a combination of a clinical risk factor score and the GCT, which was administered only in the subgroup with risk factors; in addition, two threshold values for the GCT were proposed depending on the risk score value. Using this schema, about one in three women needed no GCT, while the detection rate of GDM remained around 80%. There was also a small, but significant, reduction of false positive screening tests (i.e., an abnormal screening test but subsequent normal OGTT), from 17.9 to 15.4% of all tests. However, as the editorialist to this paper pointed out, "despite its scientific merits, busy obstetricians are unlikely to wend their way through this complex diagnostic schema for each pregnant woman".

The GCT value is known to be dependent on the time since the last meal: the so-called "Staub-Traugott" effect. Sermer et al [21] analyzed the results of 4254 GCTs, and confirmed that 1-hour plasma glucose values show a U-shaped curve depending on the time since the last meal: the lowest glucose levels were observed with the last meal 1-2 hours before. On the basis of receiver-operator characteristic (ROC) curve analysis, the following plasma glucose cut-off values were proposed: 8.2 (148 mg/dl), 7.9 (142 mg/dl) and 8.3 mmol/l (150 mg/dl) for elapsed postprandial times of <2, 2-3, and >3 hours, respectively. Using these GCT criteria and subsequently using the NDDG criteria for the OGTT diagnostic test (see "The 3-hour 100-g OGTT"), the false-positive rate dropped from 17.1 to 12.1%.

Every abnormal GCT should be followed by a diagnostic OGTT. Carpenter and Coustan [19] and Landy et al [27] investigated whether there is a threshold value above which a OGTT would not be necessary. Carpenter and Coustan [19] performed an OGTT in 109 women with a GCT value of ≥ 130 mg/dl, and found that women with a GCT value of ≥183 mg/dl had a 95% probablility of having GDM. Landy et al [27], from 514 positive screening tests followed by an OGTT, reported that a GCT cut-off value of ≥ 186 mg/dl had a high specificity (96%) for "diagnosing" GDM. A large-scale study is needed to corroborate this conclusion.

A GCT test is recommended in all pregnancies (save low-risk women), irrespective of whether the GCT was normal or abnormal in a previous pregnancy [23]. One study found that the long-term reproducibility of the GCT (1 or 2 years interval) was comparable to the short-term reproducibility (1 day); the author calculated that women with a GCT result < 125 mg/dl would not need retesting in a subsequent pregnancy within 2 years [28]. Young et al [29] retested 381 women with a normal GCT in a subsequent pregnancy, and found that none had GDM (diagnosed after OGTT), although 45 (12%) had an abnormal GCT. This important finding needs to be confirmed in further studies.

Several practical issues have been investigated. Glucose is usually given as a lemon/lime-flavored concentrated glucose solution (50 g in 150 ml fluid) or as a cola beverage. In an effort to produce more "mother-friendly" screening tests, a more dilute glucose solution (in 450 ml fluid) and confectionery (28 jelly beans) have been tested. As glucometers become more accurate, immediate analysis at the clinic of venous (or capillary) blood glucose could be used to reduce or replace the need for using plasma glucose assays; however, at this time, laboratory analysis remains the standard.

Fasting or random plasma glucose and other measurements

The value of fasting plasma glucose (FPG) as a screen for GDM was investigated in two recent studies. From a database of about 5000 Brazilian women who underwent a 75-g OGTT between 24 and 28 weeks, Reichelt et al [30] reported that 89 mg/dl was the best FPG cut-off value to screen for diabetes [according to WHO (1980) criteria, which was found in 0.3% of women], and 81 mg/dl was the best cut-off value to diagnose IGT (found in 7.3% of women). Perucchini et al [31] compared the GCT and the FPG value during a 100-g OGTT data (the GCT was performed between 24 and 28 weeks and the OGTT within 1 week of the GCT) in a cohort of 520 women with a GDM prevalence of 10.2% (diagnosed by Carpenter-Coustan criteria, see "The 3-hour 100-g OGTT"). ROC curve analysis showed that the best cut-off value for FPG was 4.8 mmol/l (86 mg/dl), with a comparable sensitivity but improved specificity (91 vs. 76%) compared with the GCT. From these studies, it appears that a FPG level of 4.8 mmol/l or 85 mg/dl [30] between 24 and 28 weeks would be a reasonable cut-off value to screen for GDM. Whether a fasting blood sample is more or less practical than a GCT between 24 and 28 weeks of pregnancy, depends on how a particular obstetric unit is organized (in most clinics, women are now given individual appointments throughout the day).

A random plasma glucose measurement within 2 or > 2 hours of a meal has been proposed as a screening test, but several recent studies have demonstrated that the sensitivity of this measurement to screen for GDM is poor, while the false-positive rate is higher than with the GCT [32]. In addition, glycohemoglobin levels and glycated serum protein (fructosamine) levels are insufficiently sensitive to be used as a screening test, although they can be of benefit in the management of GDM.

Many practicioners are unsure on how to screen for GDM. For example, in a recent national survey in the UK, only 42% of the units had a protocol for screening for GDM [33]. This is not surprising, given the conflicting scientific data and the evolving recommendations by various colleges and societies. On the basis of current scientific evidence, the author would recommend to continue (or start) performing a GCT between 24 and 28 weeks in all pregnancies, until more data become available on GDM in specific "low-risk" groups and on the need for retesting in subsequent pregnancies. Alternatively, a FPG level can be used as a screening test between 24 and 28 weeks.

■ The diagnosis of GDM

There is consensus that, in clinical practice, an OGTT should be performed to diagnose GDM. Which OGTT and which threshold values should be used remains the object of scientific debate. In North America as well as in many continental European centers, the 100-g OGTT is the standard diagnostic test; in the British Isles and elsewhere, the 75-g OGTT – as used for nonpregnant subjects – prevails. The ADA now [23] states that both OGTTs are acceptable to diagnose GDM, reversing previous recommendations to use the 100-g OGTT. The ADA now also states that a diagnostic OGTT – without a previous screening test – may be considered in populations at high risk for GDM, on the basis of data of Pettitt et al [34] obtained in Native Americans.

Any OGTT "should be done in the morning, after an overnight fast of 8-14 hours, and after at least 3 days of unrestricted diet (≥ 150 g carbohydrate per day) and unlimited physical activity. The subject should remain seated and should not smoke throughout the test" [23]. However, recent sutdies point out that a preparatory high-carbohydrate diet is unnecessary [35].

The 3-hour 100-g OGTT

The cut-off values for plasma glucose in the 100-g OGTT, as recommended by the ADA until 1999, were obtained by conversion of whole-blood glucose values as defined by O'Sullivan and Mahan in 1964, using a 1.15 conversion factor derived from studies in nonpregnant subjects and rounded to the nearest 5 mg/dl (*table I*). If two or more values are abnormal, GDM is diagnosed. Since these cut-off values had been approved by the National Diabetes Data group in 1979, they are usually referred to as "the NDDG criteria". Data from about 1000 paired whole blood and plasma glucose measurements in pregnant women by Sacks et al [36] demonstrated that the O'Sullivan and Mahan data in pregnancy should actually be converted to: 96 mg/dl fasting, 172 mg/dl after 1 hour, 152 mg/dl after 2 hours, and 131 mg/dl after 3 hours. These values are closer to the cut-off values proposed by Carpenter and Coustan [19] (*table I*) than to the NDDG criteria; the "Carpenter-Coustan" (C-C) criteria were obtained by a different conversion calculation [plasma glucose = (whole-blood glucose – 5 mg/dl) × 1.14, rounded to the nearest 5 mg/dl]. Therefore, the ADA [23], following the recommendations of the Fourth International Workshop Conference on Gestational Diabetes Mellitus [22], now endorses switching to the C-C criteria.

To be sure, the number of women with a diagnosis of GDM increases substantially when applying the C-C criteria. In the Toronto Tri-Hospital Project (comprising 3717 women), the number of women with a diagnosis of GDM would have increased by 80% [37], in the Kaiser Permanente Northwest HMO (8857 women) by 54% [13], and in the Puget Sound HMO (2019 women) by 52% [38], if the C-C rather than the NDDG criteria would have been used. In the Toronto cohort, the group with GDM according to C-C criteria but not according to the NDDG criteria – who were labeled to have "borderline GDM" – had a significantly higher rate of macrosomia (birth weight >4 kg) than women with a normal OGTT or women with known treated GDM (i.e., positive OGTT according to NDDG criteria).

Table I. Diagnosis of GDM with a 100-g oral glucose tolerance test.

	"NDDG" criteria (National Diabetes Data Group)			"Carpenter-Coustan" criteria	
	Blood	Plasma		Plasma	
	mg/dl	mg/dl	mmol/l	mg/dl	mmol/l
Fasting	90	105	5.8	95	5.3
1 h	165	190	10.5	180	10.0
2 h	145	165	9.1	155	8.6
3 h	125	145	8.0	140	7.8

Two or more of the venous blood/plasma glucose concentrations must be met of exceeded for a positive diagnosis.

The cesarean section rate was also higher in the "borderline GDM" group than in women with a normal OGTT, as a result of the increased macrosomia rate. Studies have also shown that "one abnormal value" on the 100-g OGTT is associated with an increased macrosomia rate [39]. In fact, the macrosomia and cesarean section rate, but not the fetal trauma rate, in the Toronto study were positively correlated with maternal glucose values after a GCT or during a 100-g OGTT in 3637 women without GDM [40]. For the practicioner, the obvious question then arises whether the increased macrosomia rate in women with "borderline GDM" is clinically significant as to merit glucose monitoring and treatment of the latter group, and whether it is cost effective. As of 2000 opinions differ on the clinical significance of "borderline GDM": some groups advocate treating and monitoring these women [39], whereas others warn against overtreatment [13]. In the Toronto study, the lower macrosomia rate in treated GDM women versus women with "borderline GDM" was not translated into a lower cesarean section rate: indeed, the cesarean section rate in women with treated GDM was found to be increased independently of macrosomia, probably representing an alteration in "practice style" [37]. However, a survey from birth certificates of 1993 in South Carolina showed that GDM (prevalence: 2.9%) conferred only a moderate increase in cesarean section risk [1.7 (95% CI, 1.4-2.1)], much smaller than that of pregestational diabetes [6.2 (4.5-8.6)] [41]. In one Australian center, the age- and parity-adjusted cesarean section rate was not found to be increased in women with GDM [42].

The 2-hour 75-g OGTT

For the 75-g OGTT, different criteria are being used. In many centers, the 1985 WHO criteria for nonpregnant subjects are used, with "diabetes" and "IGT" as diagnostic categories. However, because of the pregnancy-induced changes in fasting and postprandial glucose values, these criteria are not appropriate for use in pregnant women. Indeed, reviewing several relevant studies, Cheng and Salmon [43] showed that the WHO upper limit for fasting plasma glucose is far too high for pregnant women; conversely, the 2-hour glucose value is too low. Hence, adaptations for pregnant women are mandatory. *Table II* shows the cut-off values currently endorsed by the ADA [23], following the proposal of the Fourth International Conference on GDM [22]. The values are similar to the fasting, 1- and 2-hour values of the 100-g OGTT. Two or more values must be abnormal for the diagnosis of GDM. The report mentions that "this test is not as well validated as the 100-g OGTT". Indeed, recent studies documented that 2-hour glucose values were significantly higher during a 100-g than during a 75-g OGTT [44], and that omission of the 3-hour value during the 100-g OGTT lowered its sensitivity to diagnose GDM by 13% [45]. Sacks et al [46] performed a 75-g OGTT in about 2100 women between 24 and 28 weeks: mean plasma glucose levels were 84, 128 and 108 mg/dl for fasting, 1- and 2-hour timepoints, respectively; the +2 SD levels were 101, 194 and 158 mg/dl, respectively (*table II*).

The WHO has recently lowered the fasting plasma glucose threshold to diagnose diabetes from 7.8 (140 mg/dl) to 7.0 nmol/l (126 mg/dl). Schmidt et al [47] found that this barely changed the prevalence of GDM in a Brazilian population of about 5000 women. Not unexpectedly, the lower 2-hour threshold for GDM-IGT, as compared with the 100-g OGTT, resulted in a GDM prevalence of 7.6%, 94.5% of whom had IGT and only 5.5% diabetes.

Table II. Diagnosis of GDM with the 75-g oral glucose tolerance test.

	Provisional 1998 WHO recommendations		ADA 2000 recommendations		Data from Sacks et al [46]	
	Plasma		Plasma		Plasma	
	mg/dl	mmol/l	mg/dl	mmol/l	mg/dl*	mmol/l
Fasting	126	7.0	95	5.3	100	5.6
1 h	-	-	180	10.0	195	10.8
2 h	140	7.8 (IGT)	155	8.6	160	8.8
	200	11.1 (DM)				

Two or more of the venous plasma glucose concentrations must be met or exceeded for a positive diagnosis.
DM, diabetes mellitus; IGT, impaired glucose tolerance.
*Rounded values.

It has been argued that it would be logical to use the same OGTT procedure in nonpregnant and pregnant subjects, especially in high-prevalence groups [34]. In nonpregnant subjects, carbohydrate disorders are divided into three diagnostic categories: diabetes mellitus, impaired fasting glucose and IGT. Again, it would be logical to use the same diagnostic classification in pregnant women, using pregnancy-specific cut-off values [13]. Hopefully, the investigators of the large ongoing HAPO (Hyperglycemia Adverse Pregnancy Outcome) Study, a study in about 25,000 women funded by the National Institute of Health (USA), will by 2003 be able to define diagnostic categories and thresholdvalues for the 75-g OGTT, based on the perinatal outcome (http://www.hapo.nwu.edu, password required to access site).

Medical management of GDM

After GDM has been diagnosed, most practitioners would prescribe medical nutrition therapy (MNT), encourage moderate exercise and monitor glycemic control. The principles of MNT have been outlined elsewhere [23]. The meal plan consists of three meals and three snacks, with 10-20% of calories derived from protein and <10% from saturated fats, and the rest from unsaturated fats and carbohydrate. Recently, a low-carbohydrate diet (<42%) was found to result in improved glycemic control and perinatal outcome compared with a diet containing 45-50% carbohydrate [48]. The caloric content is calculated from the patient's prepregnancy bodyweight or BMI. Moderate (33%) calorie restriction, i.e., a 1600-1800 kcal diet, reduces hyperglycemia without inducing ketonuria in obese women. On the other hand, severe (50%) calorie restriction should be avoided: a 1200-kcal diet was shown to produce a significant increase in ketonemia in obese women with GDM [49]. Urine ketone monitoring is useful to detect insufficient calorie or carbohydrate intake.

Women with GDM should be encouraged to continue or start moderate exercise programs. A program of arm ergometer training (20 minutes three times a week) with MNT was shown to be superior to MNT alone in terms of glycemic control [50]. Another study, however, found no additional effect of cycle ergometer training on glycemic control in women with GDM on MNT [51].

Self-monitoring of blood glucose (SMBG) has become the standard metabolic surveillance for women with GDM. The target value for fasting/preprandial blood glucose is <90-95 mg/dl (<5.0-5.3 mmol/l), <130-140 mg/dl (<7.2-7.8 mmol/l) for 1-hour postprandial blood glucose, and <120 mg/dl (<6.7 mmol/l) for 2-hour blood glucose. Memory-based reflectance glucometers have been found to improve patient compliance and perinatal outcome in some centers. Alternatively or additionally, some centers use (two-) weekly fasting and 1- or 2-hour postprandial plasma glucose testing at the hospital to monitor metabolic control [52, 53]. Interestingly, an identical meal given to women with GDM produced higher 1-hour postprandial glucose values in the morning (07:00 hours) than in the evening (21:00 hours); the 2-hour postprandial values were similar while 3-9-hour postprandial values were higher after the evening meal [54]. This is in line with the clinical experience that 1-h postprandial values are highest after breakfast, which may be related to increased cortisol levels in the morning. In women with elevated glycohemoglobin or fructosamine levels at diagnosis of GDM, regular follow-up measurements are recommended to confirm SMBG measurements.

Human insulin preparations should be added to the treatment plan, when SMBG data show unsatisfactory glycemic control by the above measures. In women with severe fasting hyperglycemia [White class B_1, i.e., FPG $\geq$ 130 mg/dl (7.2 mmol/l)] – which constitutes a diagnosis of true diabetes very likely to persist after delivery – immediate insulin therapy is warranted. Some practitioners would also include insulin in the treatment plan from diagnosis in women with moderate fasting hyperglycemia [White class A_2, i.e., FPG 105-129 mg/dl]. It was recently shown that women with a FPG level >95 mg/dl (5.3 mmol/l) are more likely to need insulin for satisfactory glycemic control [55]. de Veciana et al [53] reported that guiding the treatment on 1-hour postprandial rather than preprandial glucose monitoring increased the insulin requirement but improved glycemic control and perinatal outcome; other groups found that adding 2-hour postprandial plasma glucose testing in addition to FPG measurements was of little significance on perinatal outcome [52]. Fetal macrosomia, as detected by ultrasound measurement of the abdominal circumference, or fetal hyperinsulinemia detected by amniotic fluid insulin measurement, early in the third trimester may constitute additional indications for adding insulin to the treatment plan in women without fasting hyperglycemia. Overaggressive treatment of GDM with insulin should be avoided, as this increases the risk of small-for-gestational-age babies [56]. Intermediate-acting insulin (once or twice daily), or a combination of rapid- and intermediate-acting insulin (before meals and at bedtime, respectively) can be used, depending to the severity of the hyperglycemia. Short-term use of human insulin preparations still induces insulin antibodies in about 50% of women with GDM, which disappear gradually after delivery [57]. In a preliminary trial, insulin lispro, a rapid-acting insulin analog that can be injected just before meals, has been shown to reduce glucose and insulin areas under the curve during a meal test in women with GDM, and to reduce the number of hypoglycemic episodes [58]; however, insulin analogs are not recommended for use in pregnant women until more safety data become available.

There is a renewed interest in the use of oral hypoglycemic agents in women with GDM, particularly in areas with a high prevalence of obese GDM women, in developing countries, etc. Older sulfonylurea drugs are not recommended, because of potential teratogenicity and a higher risk of adverse perinatal outcome. However, the potential use of metformin during pregnancy is now again being investigated, although not as yet for women with GDM. Newer oral hypoglycemic agents have also been studied. Langer et al [59] showed that glyburide does not cross the placenta. They compared the use of glyburide in women with GDM after 11 weeks of pregnancy with that of insulin (about 200 women each): glyburide and insulin resulted in comparable glycemic control (albeit with less hypoglycemic values for glyburide) and a comparable perinatal outcome.

References

[1] Catalano PM, Tyzbir ED, Roman NM, Amini SB, Sims EAH. Longitudinal changes in insulin release and insulin resistance in nonobese pregnant women. *Am J Obstet Gynecol* 1991; 165(6 (Pt. 1)): 1667-1672.

[2] Xiang AH, Peters RK, Trigo E, Kjos SL, Lee WP, Buchanan TA. Multiple metabolic defects during late pregnancy in women at high risk for type 2 diabetes. *Diabetes* 1999; 48(4): 848-854.

[3] Caruso A, Ferrazzani S, De Carolis S, Lucchese A, Lanzone A, Paradisi G. Carbohydrate metabolism in gestational diabetes: effect of chronic hypertension. *Obstet Gynecol* 1999; 94(4): 556-561.

[4] McEvoy RC, Franklin B, Ginsberg-Fellner F. Gestational diabetes mellitus: evidence for autoimmunity against the pancreatic beta cells. *Diabetologia* 1991; 34: 507-510.

[5] Füchtenbusch M, Ferber K, Standl E, Ziegler A-G. Prediction of type 1 diabetes postpartum in patients with gestational diabetes mellitus by combined islet cell autoantibody screening. A prospective multicenter study. *Diabetes* 1997; 46(9): 1459-1467.

[6] Solomon CG, Willett WC, Carey VJ, Rich-Edwards J, Hunter DJ, Colditz GA et al. A prospective study of pregravid determinants of gestational diabetes mellitus. *JAMA* 1997; 278(13): 1078-1083.

[7] Aberg A, Rydhstroem H, Frid A. Impaired glucose tolerance associated with adverse pregnancy outcome: a population-based study in southern Sweden. *Am J Obstet Gynecol* 2001; 184(1): 77-83.

[8] Branchtein L, Schmidt MI, Mengue SS, Reichelt ÂJ, Matos MCG, Duncan BB. Waist circumference and waist-to-hip ratio are related to gestational glucose tolerance. *Diabetes Care* 1997; 20(4): 509-511.

[9] Dornhorst A, Paterson CM, Nicholls JSD, Wadsworth J, Chiu DC, Elkeles RS et al. High prevalence of gestational diabetes in women from ethnic minority groups. *Diabetic Med* 1992; 9: 820-825.

[10] Naylor CD, Sermer M, Chen E, Farine D. Selective screening for gestational diabetes mellitus. *N Engl J Med* 1997; 337(22): 1591-1596.

[11] Jang HC, Min HK, Lee HK, Cho NH, Metzger BE. Short stature in Korean women: a contribution to the multifactorial predisposition to gestational diabetes mellitus. *Diabetologia* 1998; 41: 778-783.

[12] Holte J, Gennarelli G, Wide L. High prevalence of polycystic ovaries and associated clinical, endocrine, and metabolic features in women with previous gestational diabetes mellitus. *J Clin Endocrinol Metab* 1998; 83(4): 1143-1150.

[13] Schwartz DB, Daoud Y, Zazula P, Goyert G, Bronsteen R, Wright D et al. Gestational diabetes mellitus: metabolic and blood glucose parameters in singleton versus twin pregnancies. *Am J Obstet Gynecol* 1999; 181(4): 912-914.

[14] Joffe GM, Esterlitz JR, Levine RJ, Clemens JD, Ewell MG, Sibai BM et al. The relationship between abnormal glucose tolerance and hypertensive disorders of pregnancy in healthy nulliparous women. *Am J Obstet Gynecol* 1998; 179(4): 1032-1037.

[15] Fisher JE, Smith RS, Lagrandeur R, Lorenz RP. Gestational diabetes mellitus in women receiving beta-adrenergics and corticosteroids for threatened preterm delivery. *Obstet Gynecol* 1997; 90(6): 880-883.

[16] Landy HJ, Isada NB, McGinnis J, Ratner R, Grossman JH. The effect of chronic steroid therapy on glucose tolerance in pregnancy. *Am J Obstet Gynecol* 1988; 159(3): 612-615.

[17] Griffin ME, Coffey M, Johnson H, Scanlon P, Foley M, Stronge J et al. Universal vs. risk factor-based screening for gestational diabetes mellitus: detection rates, gestation at diagnosis and outcome. *Diabetic Med* 2000; 17: 26-32.

[18] Engelgau MM, Herman WH, Smith PJ, German RR, Aubert RE. The epidemiology of diabetes and pregnancy in the U.S., 1988. *Diabetes Care* 1995; 18(7): 1029-1033.

[19] Carpenter MW, Coustan DR. Criteria for screening tests for gestational diabetes. *Am J Obstet Gynecol* 1982; 144(7): 768-773.

[20] Bonomo M, Gandini ML, Mastropasqua A, Begher C, Valentini U, Faden D et al. Which cutoff level should be used in screening for glucose intolerance in pregnancy? *Am J Obstet Gynecol* 1998; 179(1): 179-185.

[21] Sermer M, Naylor CD, Gare DJ, Kenshole AB, Ritchie JWK, Farine D et al. Impact of time since last meal on the gestational glucose challenge test. The Toronto Tri-Hospital Gestational Diabetes Project. *Am J Obstet Gynecol* 1994; 171(3): 607-616.

[22] Metzger BE, Coustan DR. Summary and recommendations of the Fourth International Workshop-Conference on gestational diabetes mellitus. *Diabetes Care* 1998; 21(suppl 2): B161-B167.

[23] American Diabetes Association. Gestational diabetes mellitus. *Diabetes Care* 2000; 23(suppl 1): S77-S79.

[24] Williams CB, Iqbal S, Zawacki CM, Yu D, Brown MB, Herman WH. Effect of selective screening for gestational diabetes. *Diabetes Care* 1999; 22(3): 418-421.

[25] Moses RG, Moses J, Davis WS. Gestational diabetes: do lean young Caucasian women need to be tested? *Diabetes Care* 1998; 21(3): 1803-1806.

[26] Lemen PM, Wigton TR, Miller-McCarthey AJ, Cruikshank DP. Screening for gestational diabetes in adolescent pregnancies. *Am J Obstet Gynecol* 1998; 178(6): 1251-1256.

[27] Landy HJ, Gómez-Marín O, O'Sullivan MJ. Diagnosing gestational diabetes mellitus: use of a glucose screen without administering the glucose tolerance test. *Obstet Gynecol* 1996; 87(3): 395-400.

[28] Phillipov G. Short- and long-term reproducibility of the 1-h 50-g glucose challenge test. *Clin Chem* 1996; 42(2): 255-257.

[29] Young C, Kuehl TJ, Sulak PJ, Allen SR. Gestational diabetes screening in subsequent pregnancies of

previously healthy patients. *Am J Obstet Gynecol* 2000; 182(5): 1024-1026.

[30] Reichelt AJ, Spichler ER, Branchtein L, Nucci LB, Franco LJ, Schmidt MI. Fasting plasma glucose is a useful test for the detection of gestational diabetes. *Diabetes Care* 1998; 21(8): 1246-1249.

[31] Perucchini D, Fischer U, Spinas GA, Huch R, Huch A, Lehmann R. Using fasting plasma glucose concentrations to screen for gestational diabetes mellitus: prospective population based study. *BMJ* 1999; 319: 812-815.

[32] McElduff A, Goldring J, Gordon P, Wyndham L. A direct comparison of the measurement of a random plasma glucose and a post-50g glucose load glucose, in the detection of gestational diabetes. *Aust NZ J Obstet Gynaecol* 1994; 34(1): 28-30.

[33] Aldrich CJ, Moran PA, Gillmer MDG. Screening for gestational diabetes in the United Kingdom: a national survey. *J Obstet Gynaecol* 1999; 19(6): 575-579.

[34] Pettitt DJ, Bennett PH, Hanson RL, Narayan KMV, Knowler WC. Comparison of World Health Organization and National Diabetes Data Group procedures to detect abnormalities of glucose tolerance during pregnancy. *Diabetes Care* 1994; 17(11): 1264-1268.

[35] Crowe SM, Mastrobattista JM, Monga M. Oral glucose tolerance test and the preparatory diet. *Am J Obstet Gynecol* 2000; 182(5): 1052-1054.

[36] Sacks DA, Abu-Fadil S, Greenspoon JS, Fotheringham N. Do the current standards for glucose tolerance testing in pregnancy represent a valid conversion of O'Sullivan's original criteria? *Am J Obstet Gynecol* 1989; 161(3): 638-641.

[37] Naylor CD, Sermer M, Chen E, Sykora K. Cesarean delivery in relation to birth weight and gestational glucose tolerance: pathophysiology or practice style? *JAMA* 1996; 275: 1165-1170.

[38] Magee MS, Walden CE, Benedetti TJ, Knopp RH. Influence of diagnostic criteria on the incidence of gestational diabetes and perinatal morbidity. *JAMA* 1993; 269(5): 609-615.

[39] Langer O, Brustman L, Anyaegbunam A, Mazze R. The significance of one abnormal glucose test value on adverse outcome in pregnancy. *Am J Obstet Gynecol* 1987; 157(3): 758-763.

[40] Sermer M, Naylor CD, Gare DJ, Kenshole AB, Ritchie JWK, Farine D. Impact of increasing carbohydrate intolerance on maternal-fetal outcomes in 3637 women without gestational diabetes. *Am J Obstet Gynecol* 1995; 173(1): 146-156.

[41] Remsberg KE, McKeown RE, McFarland KF, Irwin LS. Diabetes in pregnancy and cesarean delivery. *Diabetes Care* 1999; 22(9): 1561-1567.

[42] Moses RG, Knights SJ, Lucas EM, Moses M, Russell KG, Coleman KJ et al. Gestational diabetes: is a higher cesarean section rate inevitable? *Diabetes Care* 2000; 23(1): 15-17.

[43] Cheng L-C, Salmon YM. Are the WHO (1980) criteria for the 75 g oral glucose tolerance test appropriate for pregnant women? *Br J Obstet Gynaecol* 1993; 100(7): 645-648.

[44] Weiss PAM, Haeusler M, Kainer F, Pürstner P, Haas J. Toward universal criteria for gestational diabetes: relationships between seventy-five and one hundred gram glucose loads and between capillary and venous glucose concentrations. *Am J Obstet Gynecol* 1998; 178(4): 830-835.

[45] Atilano LC, Lee-Parritz A, Lieberman E, Cohen AP, Barbieri RL. Alternative methods of diagnosing gestational diabetes mellitus. *Am J Obstet Gynecol* 1999; 181(5 (Pt. 1)): 1158-1161.

[46] Sacks DA, Greenspoon JS, Abu-Fadil S, Henry HM, Wolde-Tsadik G, Yao JFF. Toward universal criteria for gestational diabetes: the 75-gram glucose tolerance test in pregnancy. *Am J Obstet Gynecol* 1995; 172(2 (Pt. 1)): 607-614.

[47] Schmidt MI, Matos MC, Reichelt AJ, Costa Forti A, de Lima L, Duncan BB. Prevalence of gestational diabetes mellitus-do the new WHO criteria make a difference? *Diabetic Med* 2000; 17: 376-380.

[48] Major CA, Henry J, De Veciana M, Morgan MA. The effects of carbohydrate restriction in patients with diet-controlled gestational diabetes. *Obstet Gynecol* 1998; 91(4): 600-604.

[49] Magee MS, Knopp RH, Benedetti TJ. Metabolic effects of 1200-kcal diet in obese pregnant women with gestational diabetes. *Diabetes* 1990; 39(2): 234-240.

[50] Jovanovic-Peterson L, Durak EP, Peterson CM. Randomized trial of diet versus diet plus cardiovascular conditioning on glucose levels in gestational diabetes. *Am J Obstet Gynecol* 1989; 161(2): 415-419.

[51] Avery MD, Leon AS, Kopher RA. Effects of a partially home-based exercise program for women with gestational diabetes. *Obstet Gynecol* 1997; 89(1): 10-15.

[52] Huddleston JF, Cramer MK, Vroon DH. A rationale for omitting two-hour postprandial glucose determinations in gestational diabetes. *Am J Obstet Gynecol* 1993; 169(2 (Pt. 1)): 257-264.

[53] de Veciana M, Major CA, Morgan MA, Asrat T, Toohey JS, Lien JM et al. Postprandial versus preprandial blood glucose monitoring in women with gestational diabetes mellitus requiring insulin therapy. *N Engl J Med* 1995; 333(19): 1237-1241.

[54] Sacks DA, Chen W, Wolde-Tsadik G, Buchanan TA. When is fasting really fasting? The influence of time of day, interval after a meal, and maternal body mass on maternal glycemia in gestational diabetes. *Am J Obstet Gynecol* 1999; 181(4): 904-911.

[55] McFarland MB, Langer O, Conway DL, Berkus MD. Dietary therapy for gestational diabetes: how long is long enough? *Obstet Gynecol* 1999; 93(6): 978-982.

[56] Langer O, Levy J, Brustman L, Anyaegbunam A, Merkatz R, Divon M. Glycemic control in gestational diabetes- how tight is tight enough: small for gestational age versus large for gestational age? *Am J Obstet Gynecol* 1989; 161(3): 646-653.

[57] Balsells M, Corcoy R, Mauricio D, Morales J, García-Patterson Á, Carreras G et al. Insulin antibody response to a short course of human insulin therapy in women with gestational diabetes. *Diabetes Care* 1997; 20(7): 1172-1175.

[58] Jovanovic L, Ilic S, Pettitt DJ, Hugo K, Gutierrez M, Bowsher RR et al. Metabolic and immunologic effects of insulin lispro in gestational diabetes. *Diabetes Care* 1999; 22(9): 1422-1427.

[59] Langer O, Conway DL, Berkus MD, Xenakis EM-J, Gonzales O. A comparison of glyburide and insulin in women with gestational diabetes mellitus. *N Engl J Med* 2000; 343(16): 1134-1138.

[60] Schwartz ML, Ray WN, Lubarsky SL. The diagnosis and classification of gestational diabetes mellitus: is it time to change our tune? *Am J Obstet Gynecol* 1999; 180(6 (Pt. 1)): 1560-1571.

Chapter 2

The inheritance and development of diabetes mellitus

Donald W.M. Pearson, Alison Ross

Donald W.M. Pearson, Consultant Physician and Honorary Senior Lecturer
Alison Ross, Clinical Tutor
Aberdeen Royal Infirmary and the University of Aberdeen.

The inheritance and development of diabetes mellitus

Donald W.M. Pearson, Alison Ross

Abstract.–The term diabetes mellitus (DM) encompasses a broad group of clinical and biochemical syndromes. The condition is characterised by chronic hyperglycaemia that can result from abnormalities in insulin secretion, insulin resistance or a combination of both. The most common types of diabetes are type 1 and type 2 diabetes mellitus. Although type 1 DM usually presents in childhood or young adults, it can present at any age. The hallmark is insulin deficiency due to autoimmune pancreatic beta cell destruction in a genetically susceptible individual who has been exposed to an environmental insult. Such patients are prone to ketoacidosis and once diagnosed should be treated with insulin as a matter of urgency. Multiple loci throughout the genome are linked with the development of type 1 DM and abnormalities in the humoral and cellular immune systems, probably initiated by environmental factors, are recognised.

In contrast, most people with type 2 DM present in middle or old age and many are obese. Peripheral insulin resistance combined with a relative insulin deficiency accounts for the pathogenesis. Beta cell dysfunction has been attributed to genetic mutations, fetal malnutrition resulting in impaired beta cell development and accumulation of islet cell amyloid. Insulin resistance is recognised in many clinical situations of which obesity is the most common. Worldwide over the next decade increased longevity, greater obesity and less physical activity will be associated with a dramatic increase in the number of people with type 2 diabetes.

Keywords: diabetes mellitus, genetics, environment.

The diagnosis of diabetes mellitus (DM)

The diagnosis of diabetes mellitus (DM) must be considered in the context of a history detailing the classical symptoms of thirst, polyuria and weight loss. The blood glucose level is often clearly elevated so that a single laboratory measurement will confirm the diagnosis and indicate the need for urgent assessment and management. On the other hand, chronic hyperglycaemia is recognised in the absence of classical osmotic symptoms and in such asymptomatic individuals, early recognition of the condition is important to influence the development of the long-term complications associated with diabetes. The WHO has now published a "revised" definition, diagnosis and classification of diabetes mellitus and this will be used in this chapter.

In the presence of classical symptoms of diabetes mellitus, a venous plasma glucose of $\geq$ 11.1 mmol/l or a fasting plasma glucose concentration of $\geq$ 7 mmol/l makes the diagnosis. If there is uncertainty a plasma glucose concentration $\geq$ 11.1 mmol/l 2 hours after 75 g of anhydrous glucose in an oral glucose tolerance (OGTT) test confirms the diagnosis.

With no symptoms the diagnosis requires two abnormal glucose results, i.e., at least one additional glucose result on two separate days with a value in the diabetic range. This can be fasting or random or 2 hours following a standard glucose load. *Table I* summarises the diagnostic criteria for diabetes mellitus and *table II* the interpretation of a 75-g oral glucose tolerance test.

Table I. Diagnostic criteria for diabetes mellitus – WHO 2000 (plasma glucose mmol/l) result.

Fasting venous	Capillary	Random venous	Capillary	Comment
$\geq$ 7.0	$\geq$ 7.0	$\geq$ 11.1	$\geq$ 12.2	Diabetes confirmed
		5.5 < 11.1	6.5 < 12.2	Check fasting glucose
$\geq$ 6.1 < 7.0	$\geq$ 6.1 < 7.0			Impaired fasting glucose (IFG) – 75 g OGTT required
5.5 < 7.0	5.5 < 7.0			75 g OGTT required
$\leq$ 5.5	$\leq$ 5.5	$\leq$ 5.5	$\leq$ 6.5	Diabetes unlikely

Table II. Interpretation of 75 g oral glucose tolerance test (WHO 2000).

	Glucose (mmol/l)	Fasting		2 hour
Diabetes mellitus				
Venous	Plasma			$\geq$ 11.1
Capillary	Plasma			$\geq$ 12.2
Impaired glucose tolerance				
Venous	Plasma	< 7.0	*and*	$\geq$ 7.8, < 11.1
Capillary	Plasma	< 7.0	*and*	$\geq$ 8.9, < 12.2

The classification of DM

The WHO are encouraging the use of the terms type 1 and type 2 diabetes mellitus (*table III*). In clinical practice this encompasses the vast majority of people with diabetes mellitus although a small percentage have secondary or other types of diabetes.

The inheritance and development of type 1 DM

■ Clinical case history

Claire is a delightful 14-year-old girl who presented to her general practitioner complaining of a 2-week history of extreme thirst, increased urinary frequency and urinary volume with nocturia four times per night. Over the previous month she has lost 5 kg in weight although her appetite has been normal. She has not been dieting. Her medical history is unremarkable and there is no family history of note. She lives with her parents, brother and sister who are all well. She attends the local school, and there is no history of smoking, alcohol intake or recreational drug use. Clinical examination reveals dry mucous membranes and is otherwise unremarkable. Urine testing shows heavy glycosuria and ketonuria. A random glucose of 23 mmol/l confirms a diagnosis of type 1 diabetes mellitus.

Claire and her parents cope well with the diagnosis and after several educational sessions she is managing her diabetes effectively with self-administration of insulin, home blood glucose monitoring and significant changes in her diet. At the first return appointment to the diabetes centre she and her parents may reasonably ask for an explanation regarding the development of this condition which has had such an impact on her lifestyle and could adversely affect her reproductive and long-term health.

The following section should help clinicians answer some of her and her parents' questions. The simplest response is to explain our very limited understanding due to the impossibility of molecular, immunological or histological examination of the beta cells in the pancreas at diagnosis.

Research tells us that the condition develops in genetically susceptible individuals who at some stage between conception and clinical presentation are exposed to one or more environmental insults. These trigger an immune response leading to the gradual destruction of beta cells in the islets of Langerhans. Current views on the genetic predisposition, environmental factors and the immune process in the development of type 1 diabetes will be discussed below. There has been an explosion of knowledge about the human genome in recent years but the progress in clarifying the mechanism whereby certain individuals are at increased risk of diabetes remains unclear.

The initial evidence for an inherited susceptibility was derived from twin and family studies. Twin studies have variously reported concordance rates among monozygotic twins between 30 and 50% (reviewed by Hawkes [1]). Two more recent population-based studies have reported even higher rates of up to 70% concordance between monozygotic twins [2, 3]. It was also noted that the risk in dizygotic twins is higher than in sibs indicating that shared intrauterine environment may be important in disease aetiology. These studies point to a very

Table III. Classification of diabetes mellitus.

- **Type 1 diabetes mellitus**

| Pancreatic islet beta cell destruction |
| Usually presents in young people <30 years old , but may occur at any age |
| Ketosis prone |
| Related to histocompatibility antigens |
| Islet cell antibodies often present at diagnosis |
| Family history of other autoimmune conditions may be found |

- **Type 2 diabetes mellitus**

| Defects of both insulin secretion and of insulin resistance |
| Usually age >30 years |
| Usually obese (80%) |
| Family history of type 2 DM common |

- **Other specific types**

Endocrine

Acromegaly	Glucogonoma
Somatostatinoma	Cushing's syndrome
Aldosteroma	Pheochromocytoma

Pancreatic

Pancreatitis (trauma, infection etc.)	Pancreatectomy
Haemachromatosis	Cystic fibrosis
Carcinoma	Fibrocalculous pancreatopathy

Genetic

| MODY types 1-5, due to monogenic defects, autosomal dominant inheritance |
| Diabetes and deafness due to mitochondrial DNA mutations |
| Down's syndrome |
| Fredrich's ataxia |
| Klinefelter's syndrome |
| Lipoatrophy |
| Retinitus pigmentosa |
| Wolfram's syndrome (DIDMOAD) |
| Diabetes insipidus |
| Diabetes mellitus |
| Optic atrophy |
| Deafness |

Drugs and toxins

| Corticosteroids |
| Thiazide diuretics |
| Nicotinic acid |
| Pentamidine |

- **Gestational diabetes mellitus**

strong genetic influence but should be interpreted with some caution as they are open to reporting bias and the results could be confounded by intrauterine and post-natal environmental factors which would be expected to be similar in most cases. As the concordance rate in monozygotic twins is less than 100% it follows that additional environmental factors or triggers are also necessary for the development of the disease.

Family studies have also provided evidence for an underlying genetic susceptibility to diabetes, although many of the early studies included both type 1 and type 2 patients. The average risk to sibs of affected individuals with type 1 diabetes is 6% [4]. However, this risk is increased in HLA identical sibs to over 10% [3].

From this evidence heredity is considered important for the development of the disease and the development of molecular genetics provides insight into this complex process. However, it should be borne in mind that only 10% of newly diagnosed patients with type 1 diabetes have a family history of type 1 diabetes although in some families the history is of type 2 diabetes mellitus in a grandparent.

Molecular genetics of type 1 DM

Multiple loci throughout the genome are linked with the development of type 1 diabetes (nominated IDDM1-17). These loci were identified by a candidate gene approach and linkage analysis in families with affected family members. This process utilises markers at known loci in the genome and tries to establish whether these more commonly co-segregate with the disease than would be expected by chance alone. This allows identification of regions within the genome, which may harbour a gene that confers susceptibility to the disease. The stronger the link, the closer the marker is to the relevant gene. There are putative candidate genes at some of these sites but in most cases the specific genes and gene polymorphisms implicated have yet to be fully elucidated. It is of interest that the majority of these loci co-localise or overlap with loci that have been linked to other autoimmune diseases and it may be that some of these loci harbour common susceptibility genes whose gene products are central to normal immune function [5].

■ IDDM 1: The major histocompatibility complex, 6p21 *(fig. 1)*

The locus which has been found to be most strongly associated with type 1 diabetes is the major histocompatibility locus (MHC or HLA locus), on the short arm of chromosome 6, at 6p21. There are two major classes of human MHC antigens, I and II. The proteins of the complement system are encoded for in the same complex and are designated class III. Each class is divided into subregions. Class I has subregions A, B and C which encode the alpha chains of the class I molecules. Class II has subregions DR, DQ and DP and each of these has at least one expressed alpha and beta chain gene. All these loci, with the exception of the DRA gene, are highly polymorphic with many different allelic variants (see *fig. 1*). Although the HLA genes are highly polymorphic, certain allelic groupings are found together more commonly than would be expected by chance,

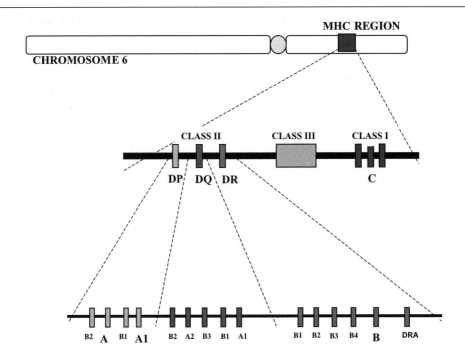

Figure 1. *A diagrammatic representation of the major histocompatibility complex on chromosome 6.*

i.e., are in linkage disequilibrium. This has complicated the identification of alleles conferring genetic susceptibility to type 1 diabetes [6].

Another cause for confusion arises from the nomenclature of the HLA class II alleles. Conventionally, the HLA molecules are now named according to the genes encoding them. The HLA molecules of the D region are prefixed by the letter "D" and then a letter denoting the sub-region, i.e., R, Q or P. This is followed by A or B denoting the alpha or beta chain. The individual alleles are denoted by a four-digit number, the first two digits of which describe the most closely associated serologic specificity. For example, the molecule previously called DQ8 is now denoted as: DQA1*0301 DQB1*0302, i.e., the molecule DQ (alpha chain 1, allele No. 0301, beta chain 1, allele No. 0302, respectively). Conventionally, an HLA-DR/DQ haplotype is named according to its DR specificity.

In 1974, susceptibility to develop type 1 diabetes was found to be associated with the class I alleles HLAB8 and B15. Later a stronger association with the class II molecules DR3 and DR4 emerged and DR3/DR4 heterozygotes were found to be at particularly high risk [7]. The previously noted association with class I alleles was secondary to linkage disequilibrium. In contrast, DR2 was rarely associated with type 1 diabetes and appeared to confer resistance.

Further studies have shown that, although DR molecules are associated with disease susceptibility, the MHC complex contains multiple susceptibility genes and alleles at the DQ locus rather than the DR locus are more closely correlated with increased susceptibility [8]. The effects of DR and DQ molecules are independent [9]. Some alleles at both the DQ beta chain gene locus and the DQ alpha chain locus have been associated with susceptibility and others have been found to confer a protective effect, however, the DQ beta locus has the major effect. Several investigators reported that the absence of an aspartic acid at position 57 of the DQ beta chain provided an excellent marker for type 1 diabetes and that the presence of an aspartic acid at this site conferred resistance [10, 11]. A subsequent study suggested that, although this was often true, it was simplistic and that only some non-aspartate alleles were associated with susceptibility [12]. It now seems that the overall MHC-linked risk is determined by the complex interactions of all the DR and DQ alleles present in an individual [9]. The haplotypes that have been associated with increased disease susceptibility and protection are summarised in *table IV*.

In conclusion, the MHC gene complex has been found to be the major locus associated with inherited susceptibility to type 1 diabetes and is estimated to account for between 36 and 50% of the inherited risk [13]. The strength of the association with the MHC gene complex is strongest in those with early onset disease [14]. The function of the MHC gene products and their putative subsequent role in the development of autoimmunity will be described later.

■ IDDM 2: The insulin gene region, 11p15.5

It is now accepted that this gene on chromosome 11 is associated with susceptibility or resistance to the development of type 1 diabetes. This gene locus accounts for a further 10% of the genetic susceptibility to type 1 diabetes [13]. Evidence of linkage for susceptibility of type 1 diabetes to a variable number

Table IV. MCH haplotypes found to confer susceptibility or protection to type 1 diabetes.

High risk			
DR3	DRB1*0301	DQA1*0501	DQB1*0201
DR4	DRB1*0401	DQA1*0301	DQB1*0302
	DRB1*0402	DQA1*0301	DQB1*0302
	DRB1*0405	DQA1*0301	DQB1*0302
Moderate risk			
DR1	DRB1*01	DQA1*0101	DQB1*0501
DR8	DRB1*0801	DQA1*0401	DQB1*0402
DR9	DRB1*0901	DQA1*0301	DQB1*0303
DR10	DRB1*1001	DQA1*0301	DQB1*0501
Protective			
DR2	DRB1*1501	DQA1*0102	DQB1*0602
DR5	DRB1*1101	DQA1*0501	DQB1*0301
DR4	DRB1*0401	DQA1*0301	DQB1*0301
DR4	DRB1*0403	DQA1*0301	DQB1*0302
DR7	DRB1*0701	DQA1*0201	DQB1*0201

tandem repeat (VNTR) sequence in the 5-prime flanking region of the insulin gene was first described by Bell et al [15]. Subsequent studies had also confirmed linkage to this locus [16].

The IDDM2 mutation was mapped to a site within the VNTR locus itself [17]. The VNTR is located within a promoter region of the insulin gene. The tandemly repeated sequences fall into three sizes. Type 1 diabetes is strongly associated with short VNTR alleles, while long repeats have a protective effect [18].

Evidence from a study by Kennedy et al [19] showed that it was likely that the VNTR sequence was involved in the regulation of insulin transcription in the pancreas and two recent studies have shown that class three VNTR alleles (high number of repeats), are associated with 2-3-fold higher insulin mRNA levels in human fetal thymus. This is where T lymphocytes undergo selection for tolerance to self-proteins. Thus, it is postulated that diabetes susceptibility and resistance associated with IDDM2 may derive from VNTR influence on the level of insulin transcription in the thymus, i.e., higher levels of proinsulin in the thymus may promote negative selection of insulin specific T lymphocytes that play a critical role in the pathogenesis of type 1 diabetes [20, 21].

■ Other loci found to be linked to susceptibility to type 1 diabetes

There is accumulating evidence in the published literature for at least a further ten loci harbouring genes implicated in susceptibility to type 1 diabetes. The sites of current interest will be briefly described here.

IDDM3 mapped to 15q26. Evidence of linkage of disease susceptibility to this locus was reported by Field et al [22] and further evidence of weak linkage was reported by Luo et al [23].

IDDM4 mapped to 11q13. Linkage of disease susceptibility to this locus has been demonstrated by several investigators [16, 24-26]. A new gene in this region has also been identified LRP5 (low-density lipoprotein receptor related protein 5), which is a possible candidate gene [27].

IDDM5 mapped to 6q25. Evidence of linkage of disease susceptibility to this locus was demonstrated by Davies et al [16] and Luo et al [23], and confirmed by Delphine et al [28].

IDDM6 mapped to 18q21. The gene for the Kidd blood group is situated in this region of chromosome 18. An association with the Kidd blood group and type 1 diabetes was described by Hodge et al [29]. Linkage of disease susceptibility to this region was confirmed by Merriman et al [30].

IDDM7 mapped to 2q31. Linkage to this region of chromosome 2 has been demonstrated by three independent groups (Refs. [16, 31]; Luo et al, 1995). Part of this region is homologous to the region of mouse chromosome 1 which harbours the murine type 1 diabetes susceptibility gene, Idd5. The region of homology may therefore harbour a similar gene, which would be a candidate in human disease. The gene for the type 1 diabetes autoantigen glutamate decarboxylase (GAD 1) also maps to the region 2q31 but this was considered an unlikely candidate gene by Copeman et al [31] as it is outside the homologous region. A further gene designated NEUROD also maps to this area and is identical to a hampster gene, which is known to regulate insulin gene expression in the hampster [32]. This gene is a further possible candidate gene for IDDM7 in humans.

IDDM8 mapped to 6q27. There is evidence of linkage to this locus on the long arm of chromosome six independent from IDDM5 [16, 23]. This was later also confirmed by Delphine et al [28].

IDDM10 mapped to 10p11-q11. Three studies have demonstrated evidence of linkage of disease susceptibility to this region of chromosome 10 (Ref. [16]; Mein et al, 1997; Ref. [33]). The gene which encodes the 65-kDa form of glutamic acid decarboxylase (GAD65), has been localised to this region but the evidence from this study suggests that this gene is unlikely to play a significant role in the genetic susceptibility of type 1 diabetes. The TCF8 gene encoding a negative regulator of interleukin 2 expression also maps to this locus and is a candidate gene for IDDM10 as interleukin 2 has a pivotal role in the regulation of T-cell function [34].

IDDM11 mapped to 14q24.3-q31. Significant linkage has also been demonstrated to this locus (Field et al. 1996).

IDDM12 mapped to 2q33. Linkage of disease susceptibility to the CTLA-4 gene in this region has been reported [35, 36]. This gene is a strong candidate gene as it encodes a T-cell receptor that mediates T-cell apoptosis and is a vital negative regulator of T-cell activation. This locus has also been associated with susceptibility to Grave's disease, another autoimmune condition [35].

IDDM13 mapped to 2q34. Linkage to this locus was described by Morahan et al [37]. Linkage to this region was also described for individuals with positive islet cell antibodies suggesting that IDDM 13 may control an early event in islet cell autoimmunity.

IDDM15 mapped to 6q21. Evidence of linkage to a third locus on chromosome 6q which was not linked to the MHC locus or the two other loci on 6q has been described [28]. Some weak support for this was also confirmed by Concannon et al [38].

IDDM17 mapped to 10q25. Verge et al [39] concluded that a locus on 10q25 was contributing to type 1 diabetes in a large Bedouin Arab family.

IDDMX mapped to Xp11. Davies et al [16] observed linkage between the X chromosome and type 1 diabetes. It is established that there is a male-female bias in type 1 diabetes and the finding of linkage to the X chromosome may explain this. Further investigation of this linkage has suggested that the male bias of patients is restricted to the HLA DR3 positive families [40].

The list of potential candidate genes will continue to expand. The future will explain the different types of genetic contribution to disease development in individuals with type 1 diabetes mellitus. In some families there are associations with other autoimmune conditions such as thyroid disease or hypoadrenalism and the genetic mechanism may be totally different from the toddler who presents with diabetes with no family history of note. Genetic make up alone does not determine the development of diabetes and it is the interplay of environment and genotype which establishes the immunological train of events ultimately leading to beta cell failure and metabolic decompensation.

Immunological abnormalities in type 1 DM

Type 1 diabetes is a consequence of insulin deficiency due to an immunologically mediated destruction of the pancreatic beta cells in genetically

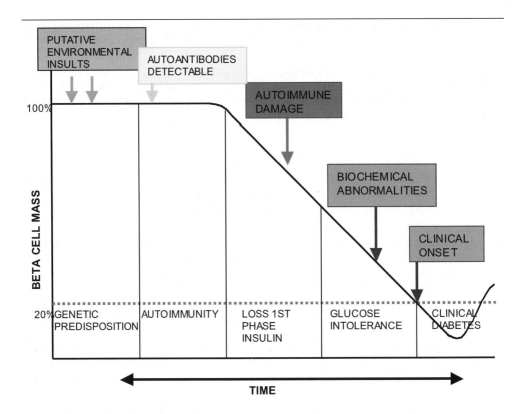

Figure 2. *Diagrammatic representation of the stages of development of type 1 diabetes mellitus.*

susceptible individuals. There is evidence from the study of first-degree relatives of cases that there is a long presymptomatic phase before the development of clinical diabetes. By the stage of overt diabetes it is estimated that over 80% of the beta cell mass has been destroyed (illustrated in *fig. 2*). Thus, the pathological process gradually destroys the beta cells over many months or years (Gorsuch et al, 1983). This finding has lead to the hope that the development of the disease may be predictable and that detection in a presymptomatic phase may allow early intervention to halt the disease process. It has also allowed further research into the pathological process itself. This process is, of course, hindered by the inaccessible nature of the beta cells of the pancreas. Biopsy or imaging studies at diagnosis are not an option! Research has therefore concentrated on changes in immune signals in the circulation.

Several abnormalities of both cell mediated and humoral immunity have been found in people with type 1 diabetes and in animal models. Autopsy specimens of pancreatic tissue of individuals who have died after presenting with diabetic ketoacidosis have shown a chronic inflammatory infiltrate of the islets of Langerhans with mononuclear cells, T and B lymphocytes and specific destruction of beta cells [41, 42]. Changes in the relative numbers of T-lymphocyte subsets in the peripheral blood of individuals with type 1 diabetes have been demonstrated and auto-antibodies to specific beta cell antigens can be detected in the peripheral blood.

However, knowledge of the pathogenic process leading to the development of type 1 diabetes remains incomplete at present. To understand the postulated mechanisms of the abnormal immune response in type 1 diabetes it is important to appreciate some of the basic principals of immunology.

■ The role of MHC molecules in the immune response

The molecules coded for by the MHC genes play a critical role in the immune response and this explains why polymorphisms in these genes may predispose an individual to the development of an abnormal autoimmune reaction.

The MHC molecules are membrane glycoproteins composed of alpha and beta chain heterodimers. Class I molecules (A, B and C), are expressed on the surface of almost all nucleated cells as well as platelets. Class II molecules have a more limited distribution and are expressed on the surface of monocytes (antigen-presenting cells), B lymphocytes and activated T lymphocytes.

The principal function of the MHC molecules is to bind antigenic peptides and present these to the cells of the immune system. Many cells in the body seem to have the capacity to fragment proteins internally and then to display peptides at their surfaces by a process involving the MHC molecules. This method of exposing the innermost cellular proteins to the cells of the immune system may allow identification of incompetent, aged, neoplastic and infected cells.

Antigen-presenting cells internalise exogenous antigens and present peptide fragments with MHC class II molecules. The MHC molecules activate T cells through binding and presentation of antigenic peptides. T cells express antigen-specific T cell receptors, which recognise specific antigen peptide sequences. There is a high degree of variability in the antigen-binding specificities of T cell receptors and to a lesser extent the MHC molecules, analogous to that for immunoglobulin chains, to allow for recognition of many antigens.

It has been found that the different sequences of the DQ gene locus alleles, particularly the codon at position 57 which usually encodes an aspartate residue, may alter the binding motifs of the MHC class II molecules. This alters the binding specificity of the binding motifs. Thus, analysis of the binding motifs in susceptible individuals may help identify the antigenic peptides responsible for triggering the autoimmune response. Signalling by the class II MHC-peptide complex is a complicated process. There is modulation of the T cell response by cytokine stimuli and accessory molecule recognition. In addition, the T cell response may also be influenced by subtle alterations in the quantity or quality of MHC-peptide expression, which are genetically determined [43].

Early studies had suggested that the MHC class II molecules were abnormally expressed on the surface of beta cells in type 1 diabetes and could thereby initiate an abnormal autoimmune response. However, this has not been verified and remains controversial.

■ The cellular autoimmune response in type 1 diabetes mellitus

The autoimmune destruction of the beta cells in type 1 diabetes is thought to be a T cell-mediated process. Evidence for this is largely derived from studies using animal models, primarily the non-obese diabetic mouse (NOD mouse). There are several groups of T-lymphocytes which have different roles and these express different cell-surface molecules. In general, helper T-lymphocytes express CD4 molecules and cytotoxic and suppressor T-lymphocytes express CD8 molecules. All T-lymphocytes also have a T cell receptor, which recognises the combination of antigen together with MHC molecules. CD4 positive cells recognise antigen presented in association with MHC class II molecules and CD8 positive cells recognise antigen presented in association with class I MHC molecules. Both of these subsets are required for the development of autoimmunity in type 1 diabetes and both have been shown to have the ability of adoptive transfer of the disease between animals. Although the specific contribution of each subset is unclear, the CD4 positive cells appear to have the major role in disease pathogenesis (reviewed in Ref. [44]).

T-lymphocytes originate from stem cells in the bone marrow but require passage through the thymus where they acquire full immunocompetence and undergo a process of positive or negative selection. This process is crucial in understanding how autoreactive lymphocytes can survive to the peripheral circulation and therefore have the potential to initiate an autoimmune response.

There have been several theories to explain a possible mechanism whereby negative selection, i.e., deletion of T cells strongly reactive with self-peptide/MHC, in the thymus may fail. Processing in the thymus has three outcomes: if there is no interaction between MHC/peptide complex and the T cell receptor then the T cells die of neglect, a low to moderate affinity interaction leads to positive selection and a high-affinity interaction leads to negative selection. Thus, there is an intrinsic production of potentially autoreactive T cells through thymic processing.

Differential avidity has been postulated as a mechanism whereby this may occur. In this model it is proposed that the avidity of the MHC/peptide and T cell interaction is crucial for both positive and negative selection and these occur at specific thresholds of avidity [45]. Avidity of the interaction is dependent on the intrinsic T cell receptor affinity for MHC, the density of T cell receptors on the lymphocyte and the density of MHC/peptide complex on the thymic antigen presenting cell. As discussed above, changes in the binding motif of the MHC molecule can alter its binding affinity for certain antigens. With diminished self-peptide/MHC binding, a compensatory increase in T cell receptor affinity would be necessary to produce the same avidity threshold for the interaction. Thus, this change in MHC molecules could allow positive selection of a population of T cells with a high affinity for self-peptides. Furthermore, in the NOD mouse the autoreactive T cells require homozygous levels of the poor peptide binding MHC for effective positive selection explaining the dominant protective effect of certain MHC alleles [43].

Although this is an elegant theory which explains the MHC association it does not explain the events by which the autoreactive lymphocytes induce disease. Animal models of autoimmunity show that while T cells with the capacity to recognise self-antigens in the periphery are a prerequisite to the development of autoimmunity their presence alone does not initiate a disease process (reviewed in Ref. [46]). Subsequent activation of such autoreactive T cells seems to involve a multi-step process [47]. This includes an amplification of T cell clones including those with autoreactivity and subsequent activation of particular T cell clones. One postulated mechanism whereby this may occur is by "molecular mimickry", i.e., a foreign antigen cross-reacts with a self-antigen leading in some individuals to the stimulation of an autoimmune reaction. The final step in the development of autoimmune disease is the failure of the usual regulatory mechanisms, such as regulatory T cells. It is likely that some of the important non-HLA genetically determined factors contribute to these last two steps which involve many complex signalling pathways [47]. From more recent data it seems likely that the autoimmune process is initiated in the pancreatic lymph nodes possibly by pancreatic islet antigen presenting cells.

■ The abnormal humoral response in type 1 DM

A number of circulating antibodies to self-antigens have been identified from the serum of patients with type 1 diabetes mellitus and also from the serum of their relatives in the prediabetic phase. These islet cell antibodies were initially detected in 80% of newly diagnosed type 1 diabetics compared with 1.5% of normal controls. These are now known to comprise auto-antibodies to a number of antigens including glutamic acid decarboxylase (GAD), and protein tyrosine phosphatase-2α and β (IA-2α, IA-2β). Antibodies to proinsulin (IAA) are also commonly detected. However, it has remained unclear whether these antigens are the primary targets of the immune response or whether they are formed as a consequence of the destruction of the beta cells [48]. It is interesting that a number of the viruses associated with the disease have antigens with sequence homology to some of the identified autoantigens thus providing some basis for the theory of "molecular mimickry" [49].

The usefulness of these auto-antibodies, as they are easily detected from peripheral blood, is as markers of the abnormal immune response and to identifiy those individuals at high risk of developing type 1 diabetes. The detection of a positive auto-antibody titre does not signal the inevitable development of the disease but the likelihood increases with rising antibody titre and with the number of different auto-antibodies detectable. Therefore, detecting combinations of auto-antibodies has a higher positive predictive power. Combining this approach with genetic screening may provide a highly sensitive and specific method to identify this high-risk group on a population basis. This would then allow for targeted immunomodulatory therapy with the aim of preventing the disease in those at highest risk. The development of auto-antibodies occurs early in life and their diagnostic sensitivity decreases with age; also, the titres fluctuate over the course of the disease. The most appropriate timing for such screening therefore still remains to be established [50].

Many questions are unanswered about the causes of type 1 DM. Knowledge has increased about the genetic and environmental interplay with immune mechanisms but considerable research is still necessary to shed light on the pathological process.

Environmental factors in type 1 DM

The incidence of clinical presentation has been shown to vary throughout the year. In summer and autumn the incidence is higher than in winter and springtime. The incidence of type 1 diabetes is increasing rapidly in many parts of the western world, most apparently in Scandinavia. Epidemiological studies have identified risk factors including a cold environment, a high growth rate, infections and stressful life events. Risk factors, which have been postulated to activate the autoimmune process, include early exposure to cow's milk proteins, nitrosamines or early fetal events such as blood group incompatibility or fetal viral infections. Epidemiological studies examining newly diagnosed and recent onset people with type 1 diabetes have suggested a role for viruses in the pathogenic process. Enteroviruses and particular coxsackie viruses B3 and B4 have been implicated since B4 can cause diabetes in animals. The time of the viral exposure to the beta cell may be important. The crucial period may be during fetal life rather than around the time of clinical presentation. For this reason, it has been very difficult to establish a clear link between a viral infection and the pathogenesis of type 1 diabetes mellitus. It is well recognised that rubella embryopathy is associated with a high prevalence of type 1 diabetes mellitus. Prospective studies performed in animals confirm that enteroviruses may initiate the beta cell destruction leading to type 1 diabetes.

Inheritance and development of type 2 DM

■ Case history

Fraser, a 64-year-old man presents with a leg ulcer that had initially occurred following trauma to the leg but has been very slow to heal. On direct questioning he has had a 12-month history of increased thirst and nocturia four times per night, which he attributed to prostate problems. He has a previous medical history of hypertension and a myocardial infarction 6 years ago from which he has made a good recovery and now only gets occasional angina. Both his sister and father have diabetes. On examination he is overweight with a BMI of 31 and there is evidence of peripheral neuropathy affecting both feet. His random blood glucose checked by his G.P. is 25 mmol/l confirming the diagnosis of diabetes. He has come to terms with his diagnosis and is managing his diabetes with dietary modification and weight loss. He attends the diabetes centre and asks, in view of the family history of diabetes, whether his own two daughters are at risk of developing the disease later in life.

The transition from a rural and active lifestyle to the sedentary and over-nourished lifestyle in the developing and in the developed world has been associated with a dramatic increase in type 2 diabetes mellitus. People with type 2 diabetes may or may not have hyperosmolar symptoms but all cases must be recognised because of the increased risk of microvascular and, in particular, macrovascular disease. "Mild diabetes" does not exist. If hyperglycaemia is confirmed vigorous steps should be taken to optimise all cardiovascular risk factors including control of blood glucose, blood pressure, blood lipids and smoking habits.

The pathophysiological processes leading to the development of type 2 diabetes are quite different from the processes involved in type 1 diabetes and the clinical presentation of the condition reflects these differences.

Type 2 diabetes is due to a combination of impaired beta cell secretion in the context of insulin resistance. The relationship between these 2 processes is complex. Only around 20% of people with insulin resistance develop diabetes mellitus. Conditions such as acromegaly, Cushing's syndrome, obesity or long-term steroid therapy all produce insulin resistance but they are not invariably associated with diabetes suggesting that factors in addition to insulin resistance must be involved.

Beta cell function and insulin secretion in type 2 DM

Beta cell dysfunction in type 2 diabetes has been attributed to several causes. These include genetic mutations, e.g. glucose sensing defects, fetal malnutrition resulting in poor beta cell development, glucose toxicity and accumulation of islet cell amyloid.

Studies of post-mortem material in people with type 2 diabetes reveals a deposition of a proteinaceous material around the beta cells. This protein known as amylin or islet amyloid polypeptide is usually produced by beta cells as an intracellular trafficking molecule to remove proteinaceous debris. In type 2 diabetes electron microscopy of beta cells shows accumulation of amylin with a collar of the material around blood vessels and this may impair the transport of nutrients. This build up is not associated with systemic amyloidosis affecting other organs. The extent of the amyloid deposition in the beta cells relates to the severity of impaired beta cell function. In normal circumstances islet amyloid polypeptide is co-secreted with insulin and the reasons why it should build up in the beta cells of people with type 2 diabetes are not known.

At diagnosis around 60-90% of beta cell function is lost. Hyperglycaemia itself may contribute to this loss of secretion since glucose is toxic to the beta cells in high concentration. In vivo studies show inadequate beta cell secretion with relatively increased proinsulin secretion at the time of diagnosis. After diagnosis there is a continuing gradual decline of beta cell function. This provides an explanation for the clinical observation that many patients who initially achieve glycaemic control on diet alone eventually need treatment with diet and tablets or diet and insulin.

A link has been established between low ponderal index at birth and the development in later life of type 2 diabetes mellitus, hypertension and ischaemic heart disease. Fetal malnutrition, especially of amino acids, is postulated to reduce beta cell mass with a concomitant reduction in fetal growth. This permanent decrease in beta cell reserve predisposes to type 2 diabetes mellitus in later life if insulin resistance develops, for example due to obesity, the ageing process or a combination of factors.

High-risk populations can be followed prospectively to allow early identification of individuals who may eventually develop type 2 diabetes. Women with gestational diabetes come into this group and although this condition only affects between 2 and 5% of the general population, if women with GDM are followed prospectively between 20 and 50% will develop type 2 diabetes mellitus.

Insulin resistance

Resistance to the action of insulin can be measured in several clinical situations of which pregnancy and obesity are the most common. With regard to obese people a diet and exercise programme may return insulin resistance to normal but weight gain will exacerbate the problem. Only a percentage of individuals with insulin resistance develop diabetes and insulin resistance may not effect all insulin sensitive tissues. An understanding of the diverse metabolic effects of insulin provides some explanation for these findings.

The hormone insulin is involved in the control of a host of metabolic processes including nutrient uptake (e.g., glucose transport), decreased glycogen breakdown, fat synthesis, inhibition of lipolysis, protein synthesis, cholesterol synthesis and glycogen synthesis! Thus while diabetes is characterised by hyperglycaemia the importance of insulin in the regulation of growth, differentiation, anti-apoptosis, fat and protein metabolism needs to be recognised.

At a molecular level insulin has an impact on numerous metabolic pathways. It binds to a specific receptor to initiate a cascade of intracellular events in liver, muscle, fat and the beta cells. The insulin receptors are transmembrane proteins made up of two alpha sub units and two beta subunits. The hormone-binding site of the insulin receptor is outside the cell membrane where the two alpha molecules form a cradle for insulin. The two beta subunits of the insulin receptor cross the membrane and have tyrosin kinase activity. Binding of the hormone to the receptor causes a conformational change in the structure of the molecule and this initiates a series of reactions on the beta chains and inside the cell. Phosphorylation of the receptor occurs and there is also phosphorylation of intracellular insulin receptor substrates (IRS) along which the signal is passed. Several different insulin receptor substrates have been identified in different cells.

At a cellular level the action of insulin after receptor binding varies depending on the type of cell which has characteristic intracellular enzymic pathways. For example, in muscle cells insulin has key effects on stimulating glucose uptake in muscle and muscle glycogen synthesis, but this is reduced in people with type 2 diabetes. Such pathways include the uptake of glucose by the GLUT 4 transport protein, intracellular phosphorylation of glucose to glucose 6 phosphate and then involvement of the glycogen synthase complex to synthesise glycogen. Molecular pathways are also influenced by the impact of other metabolic substrates such as free fatty acids, which can contribute to insulin resistance. High free fatty acid levels have a direct effect on glucose transport but effects on post-receptor pathways have also been discovered.

Metabolism in the liver depends on regulation by insulin. In the fasting state the liver maintains the blood glucose level by a combination of glycogenolysis and gluconeogenesis. The raised fasting glucose level noted in type 2 diabetes is due to an increased in gluconeogenesis. Other factors, however, will also influence the fasting glucose level, e.g., muscle glucose uptake and free fatty acid levels. During feeding and exercise multiple metabolic pathways come into play, thus a host of genes could be involved in the development of impaired insulin secretion, insulin resistance and eventual diabetes mellitus.

From the above discussion it is apparent that many specific genes could be involved in specific signal transduction abnormalities and that these could contribute to insulin resistance or reduced insulin secretion.

Genetics of type 2 DM

In type 2 diabetes, like type 1, there is also evidence of a genetic predisposition to the development of the disease. This again comes from twin and family studies. The risk to sibs of an affected individual is about 10% above that in the general population [51]. The results of twin studies have been conflicting. Early studies reported concordance rates between monozygotic twins at greater than 90%, however, these studies relied on self-reporting and were subject to bias [52].

A recent cross-sectional population based study from Denmark found a slight but non-significant increase in concordance for type 2 diabetes among monozygotic twins compared to dizygotic twins indicating that environmental factors are likely to be more important for the development of disease. However, they also found a significantly higher concordance rate for impaired glucose tolerance in monozygotic twins. Thus they concluded that genetic predisposition may be important for the development of abnormal glucose tolerance and that non-genetic factors may determine whether a genetically predisposed individual will develop diabetes [53]. A further cohort study of monozygotic twins showed an increase in concordance for type 2 diabetes and impaired glucose tolerance with time [51]. Therefore, the extent to which type 2 diabetes is genetically determined remains uncertain at present but the recent evidence suggests that this is significantly less than was previously believed.

The concordance rates between monozygotic twins is less than 100% implying that environmental factors are also required for the development of the complete disease phenotype. There is evidence that the disease progresses through a prediabetic phase of impaired glucose tolerance that is characterised by abnormalities in insulin secretion. The progression from impaired glucose tolerance to diabetes is not inevitable and glucose intolerance is commonly found in first degree relatives of affected patients.

Less is known about the specific gene polymorphisms that predispose to disease development than in type 1 diabetes. It is likely to be a heterogeneous condition with mutations in different genes in different kindreds or populations responsible for the inherited susceptibility. The inherited predisposition in most cases is polygenic. This has been confirmed in the G.K. rat animal model, where at least three loci are implicated. The risk of developing type 2 diabetes is not linked to the MHC gene locus. Although some studies have suggested a link to the insulin gene as in type 1 diabetes the results are conflicting.

There are two main metabolic defects in type 2 diabetes: (1) a failure in insulin secretion and (2) reduced tissue sensitivity to insulin. Genetic mechanisms are implicated in both abnormalities. Genes whose products are involved in the regulation of insulin secretion from the beta cell, the modulation of insulin action from the insulin receptor to the signalling pathways and those affecting obesity are all potential candidate genes for a predisposition to type 2 diabetes [54].

■ Specific genes

Several chromosome regions have been associated with the development of type 2 diabetes:

NIDDM 1 has been mapped to 2q in a genome wide linkage scan in Mexican Americans [55]. This has not been repeated in other linkage studies. However, the NEUROD 1 gene, which has also been proposed as a candidate gene in type 1 diabetes, maps to chromosome 2q and may be a candidate gene for NIDDM 1. Two mutations in the NEUROD 1 gene have recently been described segregating with type 2 diabetes mellitus in two distinct families [56].

NIDDM 2: Mahtani et al [57] reported evidence of linkage of type 2 diabetes to a region on chromosome 12q containing the gene responsible for MODY 3. Linkage was only evident when the families were sub-classified according to early insulin levels following an OGTT and was strongest in the group with the lowest insulin levels. It was postulated that mutations in the HNF-1α gene may be responsible for the linkage observed. Bowden et al [58] confirmed evidence of linkage to this region in a subset of families with nephropathy. Another study also demonstrated evidence of linkage to this region but sequencing of the HNF-1α gene did not identify any causative mutation [59]. An independent study failed to confirm evidence of linkage at this locus but found evidence of linkage to 12q at a locus centromeric to the MODY 3 gene [60].

NIDDM 3: Several studies have reported linkage of type 2 diabetes to chromosome 20q [58, 61-64]. These studies vary in the chromosomal markers which give the highest LOD score and it seems likely that there may be more than one gene on 20q which confers susceptibility. The gene HNF 4α on 20q is known to be responsible for one of the MODY syndromes and was thought to be a likely candidate gene. However, mutation analysis studies showed only one family from 19 to have a mutation in HNF 4α which co-segregated with the disease [65]. Ghosh et al [62] and Malecki et al [66] also found no evidence that sequence changes in this gene accounted for the linkage results that they had observed. This suggests that there may be other genes at these loci, which account for the linkage results observed. Ghosh et al [62] also showed linkage of disease to chromosome 20p suggesting there may be another gene at this locus although this will need to be confirmed by further studies. However, it should be noted that a study of a British cohort failed to show evidence of linkage to either NIDDM 2 or 3 [67]. This may be because ethnic differences occur in the genetic aetiology of type 2 diabetes or because there was no analysis of subsets of patients according to age of onset or complications as in some of the other studies.

Furthermore, another recent study demonstrated mutations in IPF-1, on chromosome 13, in three families with non-MODY type 2 diabetes which segregated with the disease (Ref. [68]; Stoffers et al, 1999). Whether this locus contributes significantly to the risk in the majority of cases will need to be established. It has also been shown that mutations in the insulin receptor substrate-1 (IRS-1), a downstream regulator of insulin signalling, is associated with insulin resistance which is more marked in obese subjects [69, 70]. It is therefore a further potential candidate gene.

As discussed above, several gene regions have been identified as harbouring possible susceptibility genes for type 2 diabetes mellitus and several candidate gene polymorphisms have been identified and this list continues to expand. The majority of these have been identified in only a small proportion of the affected individuals or families and major genetic causes of the disease have remained elusive to date. It therefore seems likely that subtle mutations in many genes involved both in insulin secretion and the insulin signalling pathways will eventually prove to be related to the inherited susceptibility to type 2 diabetes. Particular gene mutations may prove to predispose to the development of specific complications and this information could become useful in targeting specific screening or therapies to particular individuals at highest risk.

■ Single-gene defects

Some specific subtypes of diabetes have a clinical phenotype similar to type 2 diabetes and these have been attributed to specific single gene defects. These include the Maturity Onset Diabetes of the Young (MODY) types 1-5 and mitochondrial mutations. These subtypes account for a small percentage of all cases, 5 and 2% respectively but could provide clues to the genes contributing to inherited susceptibility in the majority of cases. However, as discussed above, few families with type 2 diabetes have been found to have mutations in the genes responsible for the MODY syndromes.

■ Maturity onset diabetes of the young

Classical MODY is characterised by an age of onset less than 25 years, the correction of fasting hyperglycaemia without insulin for at least two years following diagnosis, non-ketotic disease and an autosomal dominant mode of inheritance. The clinical course may be mild or asymptomatic. Patients are rarely obese and the underlying defect is in insulin secretion [71]. MODY was shown by linkage studies to be a heterogeneous disease and five separate genes are now known to cause this type of diabetes (summarised *table V*). These genes encode a variety of proteins including transcription factors and as discussed above may be candidate genes for the inherited susceptibility in diabetes mellitus type 2 in some pedigrees.

Table V. Subtypes of MODY.

MODY 1	MODY 2	MODY 3	MODY 4	MODY 5
Hepatocyte nuclear factor 4α (HNF 4α)	Glucokinase (GK)	Hepatocyte nuclear factor 1α (HNF 1α)	Insulin promoter factor 1α (IPF 1α)	Hepatocyte nuclear factor 1β (HNF 1β)
Chromosome 20q12-q13.1	Chromosome 7p15-p13	Chromosome 12q24.2	Chromosome 13q12.1	Chromosome 17cen-q21.3
Binds to HNF-1α and IPF-1 promoter, regulates HNF-1α and IPF-1 transcription	Catalyses conversion of glucose to glucose-6-phosphate	Binds to A3/A4 box of insulin gene promoter and regulates insulin gene transcription	Binds to A5, A3/A4, A2, A1 boxes of insulin gene promoter and regulates insulin gene transcription	Regulates HNF-4α gene transcription

■ Mitochondrial diabetes

For many years a maternal effect in the transmission of diabetes has been consistently observed. As mitochondrial genes are maternally inherited this suggested a possible role for mitochondrial mutations in the development of diabetes. Mitochondrial mutations have been found to account for approximately 2% of all cases of type 2 diabetes. The patients show a progressive impairment of insulin secretion and may require insulin treatment. There is a frequent assosciation with sensorineural deafness and this is termed maternally inherited diabetes and deafness syndrome (MIDD). Many different mitochondrial mutations have been described but the most common is a substitution at position 3243 [72].

Conclusion

The differences between type 1 and type 2 diabetes mellitus and between these conditions and other rarer forms of diabetes can be better understood by study of their aetiologies. The interplay of genetic make up and environmental factors can in part explain the phenotypic appearance, clinical presentation and pathophysiological abnormalities that characterise the conditions.

References

[1] Hawkes CH. Twin studies in diabetes mellitus. *Diabetic Medicine* 1997; 14(5): 347-352.

[2] Kyvik KO, Green A, Beck-Neilsen H. Concordance rates of insulin dependant diabetes mellitus: a population based study of young Danish twins. *BMJ* 1995; 311: 913-917.

[3] Kaprio J, Tuomilehto J, Koskenvuo M et al. Concordance for type 1 and type 2 diabetes mellitus in a population based cohort of twins on Finland. *Diabetologia* 1992; 35: 1060-1067.

[4] Todd JA. Genetic control of autoimmunity in type 1 diabetes. *Immunol Today* 1990; 11(4): 122-128.

[5] Becker KG. Comparative genetics of type 1 diabetes and autoimmune disease. Common loci, common pathways? *Diabetes* 1999; 48: 1353-1358.

[6] Weatherall DJ . The New genetics and clinical practice, 3rd edition Oxford University Press, 1991.

[7] Wolfe B, Spencer RM, Cudworth AG. The genetic susceptibility to type 1 diabetes: analysis of HLA-DR association. *Diabetologia* 1983; 24: 224-230.

[8] Owerbach D, Gunn S, Gabbay KH. Primary association of HLA-DQw8 with type 1 diabetes in DR4 patients. *Diabetologia* 1989; 25: 942-945.

[9] She J-X. Susceptibility to type 1 diabetes: HLA-DQ and DR revisited. *Immunol Today* 1996; 17(7): 323-329.

[10] Todd JA, Bell JI, McDevitt H. HLA-DQβ gene contributes to susceptibility and resistance to insulin dependent diabetes mellitus. *Nature* 1987; 329: 599-604.

[11] Morel PA, Dorman JS, Todd JA, McDevitt HO, Trucco M. Aspartic acid at position 57 of the HLA-DQ B chain protects against type 1 diabetes: a family study. *Proc Natl Acad Sci* 1988; 85: 8111-8115.

[12] Baisch JM, Weeks T, Giles R et al. Analysis of HLA-DQ genotypes and susceptibility in insulin dependent diabetes mellitus. *New Eng J Med* 1990; 322(26): 1836-1841.

[13] Skyler JS. Prediction and prevention of type 1 diabetes mellitus. Topical Endocrinology 1998; 10.

[14] Caillat-Zucman S, Garchon H-J, Timsit J et al. Age dependant HLA genetic heterogeneity of type 1 insulin dependent diabetes mellitus. *J Clin Invest* 1992; 90: 2242-2250.

[15] Bell GI, Horita S, Karam JH. A polymorphic locus near the insulin gene is associated with insulin dependent diabetes mellitus. *Diabetes* 1984; 33: 176-183.

[16] Davies JL, Kawagichi Y, Bennett ST et al. A genome-wide search for human type 1 diabetes susceptibility genes. *Nature* 1994; 371: 130-136.

[17] Bennett ST, Lucassen AM, Gough SCL et al. Susceptibility to human type 1 diabetes at IDDM2 is determined by tandem repeat variation at the insulin gene minisatellite locus. *Nature Genet* 1995; 9: 284-292.

[18] Julier C, Hyer RN, Davies J et al. Insulin-IGF2 region on chromosome 11p encodes a gene implicated in HLA-DR4-dependant diabetes susceptibility. *Nature* 1991; 354: 155-159.

[19] Kennedy GC, German MS, Rutter WJ. The minisatellite in the diabetes susceptibility locus IDDM2 regulates insulin transcription. *Nature Genet* 1995; 9: 293.

[20] Vafiadis P, Bennett ST, Todd JA et al. Insulin expression in human thymus is modulated by INS VNTR alleles at the IDDM2 locus. *Nature Genet* 1997; 15: 289-292.

[21] Pugliese A, Zeller M, Fernandez A et al. The insulin gene is transcribed in human thumus and transcription levels correlate with allelic variation at the INS VNTR-IDDM2 susceptibility locus for type 1 diabetes. *Nature Genet* 1997; 15: 293-297.

[22] Field LL, Tobias R, Magnus T. A locus on chromosome 15q26 (IDDM3) produces susceptibility to insulin dependent diabetes mellitus. *Nature Genet* 1994; 8: 189-193.

[23] Luo D-F, Buzzetti R, Rotter JI et al. Confirmation of three susceptibility genes to insulin dependent diabetes mellitus: IDDM4, IDDM5 and IDDM8. *Hum Molec Genet* 1996; 5(5): 693-698.

[24] Hashimoto L, Habita C, Beressi JP et al. Genetic mapping of a susceptibility locus for insulin dependent diabetes mellitus on chromosome 11q. *Nature* 1994; 371: 161-164.

[25] Nakagawa Y, Kawaguchi Y, Twells RCJ et al. Fine mapping of the diabetes susceptibility locus, IDDM4, on chromosome 11q13. *Am J Hum Genet* 1998; 63: 547-556.

[26] Eckenrode S, Marron MP, Nicholls R et al. Fine-mapping of the type 1 diabetes locus (IDDM4) on chromosome 11q and evaluation of two candidate genes (FADD and GALN) by affected sibpair and linkage-disequlibrium analyses. *Hum Genet* 2000; 106: 14-18.

[27] Hey PJ, Twells R, Philips MS et al. Cloning of a novel member of the low-density lipoprotein receptor family. *Gene* 1998; 216: 103-111.

[28] Delphine M, Pociot F, Habita C et al. Evidence of a non-MHC susceptibility locus in type 1 diabetes linked to HLA on chromosome 6. *Am J Hum Genet* 1997; 60: 174-187.

[29] Hodge SE, Anderson CE, Neiswanger K et al. Close genetic linkage between diabetes and Kidd blood group. *Lancet* 1981; II: 893-895.

[30] Merriman T, Twells R, Merriman M et al. Evidence by allelic association dependent methods for a type 1 diabetes polygene (IDDM 6) on chromosome 18q21. *Hum Molec Genet* 1997; 6: 1003-1010.

[31] Copeman JB, Cucca F, Hearne CM et al. Linkage disequilibrium mapping of a type 1 diabetes susceptibility gene (IDDM7) to chromosome 2q31-q33. *Nature Genet* 1995; 9: 80-84.

[32] Tamimi R, Steingrimsson E, Copeland NG et al. The NEUROD gene maps to human chromosome 2q32 and mouse chromosome 2. *Genomics* 1996; 34: 418-421.

[33] Reed P, Cucca F, Jenkins S et al. Evidence for a type 1 diabetes susceptibility locus (IDDM10) on human chromosome 10p11-q11. *Hum Molec Genet* 1997; 6(7): 1011-1016.

[34] Todd JA. From genome to aetiology in a multifactorial disease, type 1 diabetes. *Bioessays* 1999; 21: 164-174.

[35] Nistico L, Buzzetti R, Pritchard LE et al. The CTLA-4 gene region of chromosome 2q33 is linked to and associated with type 1 diabetes. *Hum Molec Genet* 1996; 5(7): 1075-1080.

[36] Marron MP, Raffel LJ, Garchon H-J et al. Insulin dependent diabetes mellitus is associated with CTLA4 polymorphisms in multiple ethnic groups. *Hum Molec Genet* 1997; 6(8): 1275-1282.

[37] Morahan G, Huang D, Tait BD et al. Markers on chromosome 2q linked to insulin-dependent diabetes mellitus. *Sci* 1996; 272: 1811-1813.

[38] Concannon P, Gogolin-Ewens KJ, Hinds D et al. A second generation screen of the human genome for susceptibility to insulin dependent diabetes mellitus. *Nature Genet* 1998; 19: 292-296.

[39] Verge CF, Vardi P, Babu S et al. Evidence for oligogenic inheritance of type 1 diabetes in a large Bedouin Arab family. *J Clin Invest* 1998; 102(8): 1569-1575.

[40] Cucca F, Goy JV, Kawaguchi Y et al. A male-female bias in type 1 diabetes and linkage to chromosome Xp in MHC HLA-DR3-positive patients. *Nature Genet* 1998; 19: 301-302.

[41] Atkinson MA, MacLaren NK. The pathogenesis of insulin dependent diabetes mellitus. *N Eng J Med* 1994; 331(21): 1428-1435.

[42] Lernmark A, Moller C, Kockum I, Sanjeevi C. Autoimmune endocrinopathies 3: Islet cell autoimmunity. *J Int Med* 1993; 234: 361-369.

[43] Noorchashm H, Kwok W, Rabinovitch A, Harrison LC. Immunology of IDDM. *Diabetologia* 1997; 40: B50-B57.

[44] Tisch R, McDevitt H. Insulin dependent diabetes mellitus. *Cell* 1996; 85: 291-297.

[45] Munir Alam SM, Travers PJ, Wung JL et al. T-cell-receptor affinity and thymocyte positive selection. *Nature* 1996; 381: 616-620.

[46] Ridgeway WM, Fathman CG. The association of MHC with autoimmune diseases: understanding the pathogenesis of autoimmune diabetes. *Clin Immunol Immunopathol* 1998; 36(1): 3-10.

[47] Nepom GT, Kwok WW. Molecular basis for HLA-DQ associations with IDDM. *Diabetes* 1998; 47: 1177-1184.

[48] Leslie RDG, Atkinson MA, Notkins AL. Autoantigens IA-2 and GAD in type 1 diabetes. *Diabetologia* 1999; 42: 3-14.

[49] Jones DB, Crosby I. Proliferative lymphocyte responses to virus antigens homologous to GAD65 in IDDM. *Diabetologia* 1996; 39: 1318-1324.

[50] Verge CF, Gianani R, Kawasaki E et al. Prediction of type 1 diabetes in first degree relatives using a combination of insulin, GAD, and ICA 512bcd/IA2 autoantibodies. *Diabetes* 1996; 45: 926-933.

[51] Medici F, Hawa M, Inari A, Pyke DA, Leslie RDG. Concordance rate for Type II diabetes mellitus in monozygotic twins: actuarial analysis. *Diabetologia* 1999; 42: 146-150.

[52] Hopper JL. Is Type II Diabetes Mellitus not so "genetic" after all? *Diabetologia* 1999; 42: 125-127.

[53] Poulsen P, Kyvik KO, Vaag A, Beck-Nielson H. Heritability of type II diabetes mellitus and abnormal glucose tolerance – a population based twin study. *Diabetologia* 1999; 42: 139-145.

[54] Regazzi R, Verchere CB, Halban PA, Polonsky KS. Insulin production: from gene to granule. *Diabetologia* 1997; 40: B33-B38.

[55] Hani CL, Boerwinkle E, Chakraborty R et al. A genome wide search for human non-insulin dependent diabetes genes reveals a major susceptibility locus on chromosome 2. *Nat Genet* 1996; 13: 161-166.

[56] Malecki MT, Jhala US, Antonellis A et al. Mutations in NEUROD1 are associated with the development of type 2 diabetes mellitus. *Nature Genet* 1999; 23: 323-327.

[57] Mahtani MM, Widen E, Lehto M et al. Mapping of a gene for type 2 diabetes associated with an insulin secretion defect by a genome scan in Finnish families. *Nature Genet* 1996; 14: 90-95.

[58] Bowden DW, Sale M, Howard TD et al. Linkage of genetic markers on human chromosomes 20 and 12 to NIDDM in Caucasian sib pairs with a history of diabetic nephropathy. *Diabetes* 1997; 46: 882-886.

[59] Shaw JT, Lovelock PK, Kesting JB, Cardinal J, Duffy D, Wainaright B, Cameron DP. Novel susceptibility gene for late-onset NIDDM is localised to human chromosome 12q. *Diabetes* 1998; 47(11): 1793-1796.

[60] Bektas A, Suprenant ME, Wogan LT et al. Evidence of a novel type 2 diabetes locus 50cM

centromeric to NIDDM2 on chromosome 12q. *Diabetes* 1999; 48: 2246-2251.

[61] Elbein SC, Hoffman MD, Teng K et al. A genome wide search for type 2 diabetes susceptibility genes in Utah Caucasians. *Diabetes* 1999; 48: 1175-1182.

[62] Ghosh S, Watanabe RM, Hauser ER et al. Type 2 diabetes: evidence for linkage on chromosome 20 in 716 Finnish affected sib pairs. *Proc Natl Acad Sci* 1999; 96: 2198-2203.

[63] Ji L, Malecki M, Warram JH et al. New susceptibility locus for NIDDM is localised to human chromosome 20q. *Diabetes* 1997; 46: 876-881.

[64] Zouali H, Hani EH, Philippi A et al. A susceptibility locus for early onset non-insulin dependent diabetes mellitus maps to chromosome 20q, proximal to the phosphoenolpyruvate carboxykinase gene. *Hum Molec Genet* 1997; 6(9): 1401-1408.

[65] Hani EH, Suaud L, Boutin P et al. A missense mutation in Hepatocyte nuclear factor-4α resulting in a reduced transactivation activity, in human late-onset non insulin dependant diabetes mellitus. *J Clin Invest* 1998; 101(3): 521-526.

[66] Malecki MT, Antonellis A, Casey P et al. Exclusion of the Hepatocyte nuclear factor 4α as a candidate gene for late onset NIDDM linked with chromosome 20q. *Diabetes* 1998; 47: 970-972.

[67] Frayling TM, McCarthy MI, Walker M et al. No evidence for linkage at candidate type 2 diabetes susceptibility loci on chromosomes 12 and 20 in United Kingdom Caucasians. *J Clin Endocrinol Metabol* 2000; 85(2): 853-857.

[68] Hani EH, Stoffers DA, Chevre J-C et al. Defective mutations in the insulin promoter factor-1 (IPF1) gene in late-onset type 2 diabetes mellitus. *J Clin Invest* 1999; 104(9): R41.

[69] Almind K, Bjorbaek C, Vestergaard H, Hansen T, Echwald S, Pedersen O. Aminoacid polymorphisms of insulin receptor substrate-1 in non insulin dependent diabetes mellitus. *Lancet* 1993; 342: 828-832. October 2.

[70] Pedersen O. Genetics of insulin resistance. *Exp Clin Endocrinol Diabetes* 1999; 107(2): 113-118.

[71] Winter WE, Nakamura M, House DV. Monogenetic diabetes mellitus in youth. The MODY syndromes. *Endocrinology and Metabol Clinics North Am.* 1999; 28(4): 765-785.

[72] Wollheim CB. Beta cell mitochondria in the regulation of insulin secretion: a new culprit in type II diabetes. *Diabetologia* 2000; 43: 265-277.

[73] Gorsuch AM, Lister J, Dean BM et al. Evidence for a long pre-diabetic period in type 1 diabetes mellitus. *Lancet* 1981; 2: 1363-1365.

[74] Mein CA, Esposito L, Dunn MG et al. A search for type 1 diabetes susceptibility genes in families from the United Kingdom. *Nature Genet* 1998; 19: 297-300.

[75] Thorsby E, Ronninggen KS. Particular HLA-DQ molecules play a dominant role in determining susceptibility or resistance to type 1 diabetes mellitus. *Diabetologia* 1993; 36(5): 371-377.

[76] Vyse TJ, Todd JA. Genetic analysis of autoimmune disease. *Cell* 1996; 85: 311-318.

[77] Weatherall D, Sarvetnick N, Shizuru JA. Genetic control of diabetes mellitus. *Diabetologia* 1992; 35(suppl 2): S1-S7.

Chapter 3

Preconceptional care in type I diabetes

F. André Van Assche

F. André Van Assche, MD, PhD, FRCOG, Department of Obstetrics and Gynaecology, University Hospital Gasthuisberg, K.U.Leuven, Belgium.

Preconceptional care in type I diabetes

F. André Van Assche

Abstract.—Diabetes and pregnancy need preconceptional care not only to reduce perinatal morbidity and mortality, congenital malformations and miscarriages, but also to prevent diseases in later life.

Unfortunately, a large proportion of diabetic women are not taking the benefit of preconceptional care.

It seems necessary to stress further the importance of this optimal care for the diabetic pregnancy.

Keywords: diabetes and pregnancy, preconceptional care, congenital malformations, perinatal medicine.

Introduction

At the beginning of the century a large number of diabetic patients died before the age of reproduction or were too unwell to reach conception. When pregnancy occurred, maternal morbidity and mortality were extremely high and only a few children were born alive. The discovery of insulin nearly 80 years ago was beneficial for the mother, but perinatal survival was still rare. Improvements in diabetic, obstetric and neonatal care reduced perinatal mortality, but it remained high compared to the non-diabetic pregnant mothers. The best prenatal care offered to the diabetic patient was tight diabetic control even before conception.

It is for this reason that about 20 years ago preconceptional care was started in centres taking care of pregnant diabetic women. It was a joint approach of the diabetologist and the obstetrician-gynaecologist.

The practice of preconceptional care

There is a growing evidence that tight control of diabetes before pregnancy improves fetal and maternal outcome. Education and strict management may prevent congenital malformations and early pregnancy loss [1].

Many studies have shown that congenital malformations are more numerous in infants of type I diabetic mothers and these are becoming the leading cause of perinatal morbidity and mortality [2-7]. Kucera reviewed the world literature between 1930 and 1964: the incidence of congenital malformations in diabetic pregnancies was 4.8% compared with 1.65% in normal pregnancies. Anomalies of the central nervous system, heart, skeleton, gastro-intestinal tract and genito-urinary tract are predominant [8]. Poor metabolic control and the severity of diabetes is correlated with the high incidence of congenital anomalies [3-9].

An association is also found with a high level of glycosylated haemoglobin in the first trimester of pregnancy [10]. In animal experiments, high glucose concentration in vivo and in vitro induce congenital malformations [11]. Furthermore, optimal treatment with insulin in the critical period of organo-genesis during experimental diabetes reduces the rate of fetal malformations in the rat [12].

The first study in human pregnancy showing a reduction in congenital malformations by intensive diabetic management prior to conception was from Karlsberg, Germany in 1983 [13].

The incidence of congenital malformations was 0.8% in pregnancies of diabetic women given intensive treatment prior to conception and 7.8% in those pregnancies where intensive treatment started only at 8 weeks. Studies in Europe and the USA confirmed these positive findings [14-17]. Strict metabolic control early in pregnancy reduces the number of congenital malformations at birth, but does not prevent the excess frequency at and early after conception, as is the case with tight diabetic control prior to conception [7].

The relationship between poor diabetic control before conception or early in preg-nancy and an increased rate of spontaneous abortion is not so clear. Miodovnik et al concluded that control of blood sugar is crucial around conception and in the early weeks of pregnancy to reduce the risk of an early abortion. Abortions after 10 weeks are probably due to congenital malformations [18].

Studies in diabetic rats have shown delayed morphologic and functional development of blastocysts even in the pre-implantation period; early embryonic development was also affected [19].

There is therefore no doubt that preconceptional care must be offered to each diabetic woman planning a pregnancy. The woman and her partner should be informed that in the case of severe diabetes, certainly in association with hypertension, life-threatening complications for herself and the fetus do exist and exceptionally, she should be advised not to become pregnant.

The most important goal of preconceptional care is to motivate intensive self-management in order to obtain normoglycaemia. The woman must be instructed on self-monitoring her blood glucose and must learn about diet, physical activity and an efficient insulin regimen. Only when permanent normolycaemia is achieved can the future of the conceptus and maternal health be assured.

Have we realised this optimistic view by the start of a new millenium?

Judith Steel from Edinburgh summaries her vast personal experience; it remains worthwhile to invest further in preconceptional care, but a large group of young diabetic women are not yet reached early enough to get preconceptional care [20].

Holing et al reported in 1998 that the number of planned pregnancies in diabetic women remained disappointingly low; only 41% were planned pregnancies [21]. Planned pregnancies began with lower glycohaemoglobin levels and had a more stable and higher socio-economic status.

Recently, Suhonen et al showed very clearly that efforts must be increased not only to motivate diabetic women that they are provided with preconceptional care, but this preconceptional care must realise normoglycaemia [22]. Indeed even slightly raised glycohaemoglobin levels during early pregnancy in women with type I diabetes is associated with an increased risk for congenital malformations. We therefore may stress that society and all health providers must assure that all diabetic women receive optimal preconceptional care.

A new dimension supporting preconceptional care is found in the fact that intrauterine life in a diabetic environment may also have consequences for adult life. Therefore, optimal preconceptional care is not only important to reduce perinatal morbidity and mortality, but also to improve health at older age for these offspring. These perspectives open the strategy of preconceptional care not only in type I diabetic women, but also in women with an increased risk for gestational diabetes [23].

Conclusion

There is evidence that optimal preconceptional care in diabetic women is necessary in the modern concept of perinatal medicine. Furthermore, the benefit is not only for the perinatal period, but also for later life.

However, a large proportion of diabetic women are still deprived of this preconceptional care or are still missing optimal care (normaglycaemia).

References

[1] Kitzmiller JL, Gavin LA, Gunderson E. Preconception counselling: rationale for evaluation and management of diabetes prior to pregnancy. In: Lee RV, Barron WM, Cotton DV, Coustan DR, Eds. Current obstetric medicine. St. Louis: Mosby Year Book, 1991: 1-16.

[2] Gabbe SG. Congenital malformations in infants of diabetic mothers. *Obstet Gynaecol Surv* 1977; 32: 125-132.

[3] Pedersen J. The pregnant diabetic and her newborn. Baltimore: Williams & Wilkins, 1977.

[4] Cousins L. Congenital anomalies among infants of diabetic mothers: etiology, prevention, diagnosis. *Am J Obstet Gynecol* 1983; 147: 333-338.

[5] Lowy C, Beard RW, Goldschmidt J. Congenital malformations in babies of diabetic mothers. *Diabet Med* 1986; 3: 458-462.

[6] Reece EA, Hobbins JC. Diabetic embryopathy: pathogenesis, prenatal diagnosis and prevention. *Obstet Gynecol Surv* 1986; 41: 325-335.

[7] Mills JL, Knopp RH, Simpson JL, Jovanovic-Peterson L, Metzger BE, Holmes LB et al. Lack of relation of increased malformation rates in infants of diabetic mothers to glycemic control during organogenesis. *N Engl J Med* 1988; 318: 671-676.

[8] Kucera J. Rate and type of congenital anomalies among offspring of diabetic women. *J Reprod Med* 1971; 7: 73-82.

[9] Freinkel N, Cockroft DL, Lewis NJ, Gorman L, Akazawa S, Phillips LS et al. Fuel-mediated teratogenesis during early organogenesis: the effects of increased concentrations of glucose, ketones, or somato medin inhibitor during rat embryo culture. *Am J Clin Nutr* 1986; 44: 896-995.

[10] Hanson U, Persson B, Thunell S. Relationship between haemoglobin A-1c in early type l (insulin dependent) diabetic pregnancy and the occurrence of spontaneous abortion and fetal malformation in Sweden. *Diabetologia* 1990; 33: 100-104.

[11] Rashbass P, Ellington SK. Development of rat embryos cultured in serum prepared from rats with streptozotocin-induced diabetes. *Teratology* 1988; 37: 51-61.

[12] Eriksson RS, Thunberg L, Eriksson UJ. Effects of interrupted insulin treatment on fetal outcome of pregnant diabetic rats. *Diabetes* 1989; 38: 764-772.

[13] Fuhrmann K, Reiher H, Semmler K, Fischer F, Fischer M, Glockner E. Prevention of congenital malformation in infants of insulin-dependent diabetic mothers. *Diabetes Care* 1983; 6: 219-223.

[14] Damm P, Molsted-Pedersen L. Significant decrease in congenital malformations in newborn infants of an unselected population of diabetic women. *Am J Obstet Gynecol* 1989; 161: 1163-1167.

[15] Goldman JA, Dicker D, Feldberg D, Yeshaya A, Samuel S, Karp M. Pregnancy outcome in patients with insulin-dependent diabetes mellitus with preconceptual diabetic control: a comparative study. *Am J Obstet Gynecol* 1986; 155: 293-297.

[16] Steel JM, Johnstone FD, Hepburn DA, Smith AF. Can prepregnancy care of diabetic women reduce the risk of abnormal babies? *Br Med J* 1990; 301: 1070-1074.

[17] Kitzmiller JL, Gavin LA, Gin GD, Jovanovic-Peterson L, Main EK, Zigrang WD. Preconception management of diabetes continued through early pregnancy prevents the excess of major congenital anomalies in infants of diabetic mothers. *JAMA* 1991; 265: 731-736.

[18] Miodovnik M, Mimouni F, Dignan PS, Berk MA, Ballard JL, Siddiqi TA et al. Major malformations in infants of IDDM women: vasculopathy and early first-trimester poor glycemic control. *Diabetes Care* 1988; 11: 713-718.

[19] Pampfer S, De Hertogh R, Vanderheyden I, Michiels B, Vercheval M. Decreased inner cell mass proportion in blastocysts from diabetic rats. *Diabetes* 1990; 39: 471-476.

[20] Steel JM. Personal experience of prepregnancy care in women with insulin dependent diabetes. *Aust NZ J Obstet Gynaecol* 1994; 34: 135-143.

[21] Holing EV, Beyer CS, Brown ZA, Connell FA. Why don't women with diabetes plan their pregnancies? *Diabetes Care* 1998; 21: 889-895.

[22] Suhonen L, Hiilesmaa V, Teramo K. Glycaemic control during early pregnancy and fetal malformations in women with type I diabetes mellitus. *Diabetologia* 2000; 43: 79-82.

[23] Van Assche FA, Holemans K, Aerts L. Fetal growth and consequences for later life. *J Perinat Med* 1998; 26: 337-346.

Chapter 4

Abortion and congenital malfunctions

Ulf J. Eriksson

Ulf J. Eriksson, MD, PhD, Department of Medical Cell Biology, Uppsala University, Biomedical Center, P.O. Box 571, SE-751 23 Uppsala, Sweden.

Abortion and congenital malfunctions

Ulf J. Eriksson*

Abstract.—In diabetic pregnancy increased rates of spontaneous abortion, pre-eclampsia and congenital malformations occur. It is of outmost importance to strive for optimal metabolic control in the mother during the early part of pregnancy, in order to diminish the risk of developing any of these complications. In addition, recent experimental work strongly suggests an etiological role of reactive oxygen species in the pathogenesis of these complications. Strengthening the maternal oxidative defense system by administration of antioxidative substances may therefore be of therapeutical value, and should be tested in human clinical trials.

Keywords: spontaneous abortion, pre-eclampsia, congenital malformation, reactive oxygen species.

*Address for correspondence: Professor Ulf J. Eriksson, MD, PhD, Tel.: +46 18 471 4129, Fax: +46 18 550720, E-mail: ulf.eriksson@medcellbiol.uu.se

Background

Diabetes mellitus disturbs both the maternal and fetal development during pregnancy [1-4]. Despite major advances in clinical management of diabetes during the last couple of decades, perinatal mortality in diabetic pregnancy remains around 4-5 times higher than the perinatal mortality in non-diabetic control pregnancies [1, 5]. Indeed, in type 1 diabetic gestation both perinatal mortality and morbidity are elevated, as well as the incidence of fetal malformations. We will specifically discuss the effects of the disease on the mother's well-being [6] and risk of miscarriage [7], as well as the rates of morbidity [8, 9], mortality [7] and malformation [4] of the offspring.

The pathogenic mechanisms behind the developmental disturbances in diabetic gestation are not known. Several studies have suggested, however, that the severity of the maternal diabetic state is of pivotal importance [10-12], in particular in the first trimester of pregnancy.

In recent years the concept of diabetes generating a state of oxidative stress has gained acceptance [13, 14], and there are several demonstrations of markers of oxidative stress being increased in diabetic humans [15, 16] and animals [17-19]. In a recent experimental study, the notion of a hyperglycemia-induced excess of reactive oxygen species (ROS) is given support [20]. Bovine aortic endothelial cells were exposed to high glucose concentrations and a ROS excess developed. This ROS increase was prevented by an inhibitor of electron-transport chain complex II, by an uncoupler of oxidative phosphorylation, by uncoupling protein-1 and by manganese superoxide dismutase, thereby indicating that the ROS production of mitochondria in the endothelial cells is the major effect of the increased ambient glucose concentration.

Transferring this concept of glucose-induced oxidative stress to diabetic pregnancy yields the notion that the pregnant diabetic woman may expose herself and her embryo to excess ROS, in inverse proportion to the degree of metabolic control. We will use this view as an adjunct to the understanding of several of the complications that affect diabetic pregnancy, such as increased rate of spontaneous abortion, pre-eclampsia and congenital malformations.

Spontaneous abortion

Diabetic women have an increased rate of spontaneous abortion in several studies, both when the mother has type 1 or type 2 diabetes [8, 21-23]. The risk for spontaneous abortion is clearly related to the degree of glycemic control in early pregnancy [24, 25]. Consequently, when the metabolic control is optimized, the spontaneous abortion rate is diminished [7, 12, 22].

In animal studies, an association between metabolic control, antioxidative treatment and occurrence of abortions (in rodents: resorptions) has been demonstrated repeatedly. Thus, in rodents with experimental or genetic diabetes, there are increased rates of resorption [26-29]. The increased rate of fetal resorption can be diminished by improving maternal metabolic control with insulin treatment [30, 31]. This effect can also be achieved in pregnant diabetic rodents with dietary supplementation of antioxidants such as vitamin E [32-34], vitamin C [35], a mixture of vitamins E and C [36], lipoic acid [37], and glutathione [38]. The obvious similarities in the effects on resorptions and malformations exerted by insulin and antioxidant treatment foster the conclusion that these adverse conditions share etiological components. Furthermore, it was recently reported that markers of oxidative stress were increased, and levels of antioxidants decreased, in women with a history of recurrent abortions [39].

In conclusion, since markers of oxidative stress have been found to be increased in diabetic individuals [15, 16, 40, 41], and thus in mothers [19] and offspring [18, 19] of diabetic pregnancy, this ROS excess is likely to be of etiological importance for the rate of spontaneous abortion in these women. Clinical trials aiming to diminish the oxidative stress in diabetic pregnancy will therefore be of importance for delineating the future therapeutical role of antioxidative compounds.

Pre-eclampsia

A major cause of perinatal complications is *pre-eclampsia*, which occurs 2-4 times more often in diabetic than normal pregnancy (incidence of 15-25 %) and is associated with an increased risk of prematurity and perinatal morbidity in the newborn [2]. Pre-eclampsia affects 7% of pregnant women [42] and is characterized by increased blood pressure and albuminuria in the mother, often associated with growth retardation in the offspring [43]. There is no other clinical procedure than termination of pregnancy that can prevent or delay the onset and progression of pre-eclampsia.

The etiology of pre-eclampsia is not clear. One reason for the lack of understanding of the disease is the absence of an appropriate animal model for the disease. Presently, there are numerous suggestions as to the identity of possible etiological agents. Imbalances in the nitric oxide metabolism [44, 45], altered concentration of vasoactive peptides (IL-6 [46], NKB [47]), changes in the coagulation system [48-51], endothelial dysfunction [52], shallow placentation [53, 54], disturbed lipid [55] and carbohydrate metabolism [56], are some suggestions to the etiology of pre-eclampsia.

Observations in non-diabetic pregnancy have provided strong evidence that excess ROS are involved in the pathogenesis of pre-eclampsia [57, 58]. This notion has been supported by several findings in vivo [59-65] and in vitro [66-71]. In a clinical intervention study, pregnant women with abnormal two-stage Doppler uterine artery analysis [72] were supplemented with vitamin C (1000 mg/day) and vitamin E (400 IU/day), a treatment which decreased the incidence of pre-eclampsia from 17% (placebo group) to 11% (vitamin group) [73]. Antioxidant therapy resulted in a significant reduction in occurrence of circulating markers of endothelial and placental dysfunction (PAI-1 and -2), and of elevated plasma concentrations of ascorbic acid and α-tocopherol [73]. Thus, there is ample evidence from experimental and clinical work to support the notion of excess ROS being involved in the etiology of pre-eclampsia [74], presumably interacting with some of the other etiological agents [75].

Elevated HbA1c in early diabetic pregnancy, indicating metabolic stress, has been identified as a significant risk factor that could contribute to the development of pre-eclampsia [1, 76, 77]. Diabetes nephropathy is associated with an increased incidence of pre-eclampsia, and, as recently demonstrated, with incipient nephropathy [78]. These complications are closely interrelated with variables such as maternal duration of diabetes, the presence of retinopathy and most importantly the level of glycemic control. Analyses of diabetic pregnancies show that elevated HbA1c in early pregnancy is independently associated with the occurrence of pre-eclampsia [1], and that the risk for pre-eclampsia is increased by a factor of 1.5 for each 1% increment of the initial HbA1c level [77].

In conclusion, as for the occurrence of spontaneous abortion in diabetic pregnancy, clinical trials where insulin treatment is supported with antioxidative treatment will be necessary to elucidate the exact role of this therapeutical addition.

Congenital malformations

In diabetic pregnancy *congenital malformations* represent the most important single cause of perinatal mortality or severe morbidity [7]. A large number of studies have demonstrated a significant association between poor glycemic control, as reflected by elevated HbA1c values in the first trimester of pregnancy, and congenital anomalies [10, 11, 79, 80]. A series of experimental studies in rodents indicated that elevated glucose, and other substrates such as β-hydroxybutyrate or branched-chain amino acids, led to excess ROS production which in turn exerts a teratogenic effect [81]. It was recently demonstrated that metabolic stress caused by elevated glucose levels induces increased production of superoxide by the mitochondrial electron-transport chain [20]. In vitro studies have demonstrated that addition of the scavenging enzymes SOD, catalase or glutathione peroxidase to the culture medium protects the rat embryo from dysmorphogenesis [82, 83]. Of particular importance are in vivo experiments that have shown that supplementation of antioxidants like vitamin C [35] or vitamin E [32-34] or combinations of vitamins C and E [36] to the pregnant diabetic rat markedly reduces the occurrence of fetal anomalies. It is of interest in this context that a ROS excess has also been implicated in the teratogenic process caused by phenytoin [84, 85], alcohol [86-89] and thalidomide [90, 91]. Evidently, an insight into the effectiveness of antioxidative treatment in one patient group, i.e., diabetic pregnant women, may have importance for the design of treatment regimens for other types of high-risk pregnancies.

A further indirect support of the hypothesis that excess ROS has teratogenic effects is the recent demonstration that multivitamin supplementation during the periconceptional period was associated with a significant reduction of congenital heart malformations [92].

Taken together, the time has come to perform clinical studies to evaluate the possible importance of the large body of animal data supporting a role for antioxidative treatment in diabetic pregnancy.

Conclusions

It is of outmost importance to strive for optimal metabolic control in the mother during the early part of pregnancy, in order to diminish the risk for spontaneous abortion, pre-eclampsia and congenital malformation. Furthermore, strengthening the maternal oxidative defense system by administration of antioxidative substances may show to be of therapeutical value, and should be tested in human clinical trials.

References

[1] Hanson U, Persson B. Epidemiology of pregnancy-induced hypertension and preeclampsia in type 1 (insulin-dependent) diabetic pregnancies in Sweden. *Acta Obstet Gynecol Scand* 1998; 77: 620-624.

[2] Ros HS, Cnattingius S, Lipworth L. Comparison of risk factors for preeclampsia and gestational hypertension in a population-based cohort study. *Am J Epidemiol* 1998; 147: 1062-1070.

[3] Schaefer-Graf UM, Buchanan TA, Xiang A, Songster G, Montoro M, Kjos SL. Patterns of congenital anomalies and relationship to initial maternal fasting glucose levels in pregnancies complicated by type 2 and gestational diabetes. *Am J Obstet Gynecol* 2000; 182: 313-320.

[4] Aberg A, Westbom L, Kallen B. Congenital malformations among infants whose mothers had gestational diabetes or preexisting diabetes. *Early Hum Dev* 2001; 61: 85-95.

[5] Casson IF, Clarke CA, Howard CV, McKendrick O, Pennycook S, Pharoah PO, Platt MJ, Stanisstreet M, van Velszen D, Walkinshaw S. Outcomes of pregnancy in insulin dependent diabetic women: results of a five year population cohort study. *Br Med J* 1997; 315: 275-278.

[6] Ekbom P, Damm P, Nogaard K, Clausen P, Feldt-Rasmussen U, Feldt-Rasmussen B, Nielsen LH, Molsted-Pedersen L, Mathiesen ER. Urinary albumin excretion and 24-hour blood pressure as predictors of pre-eclampsia in Type I diabetes. *Diabetologia* 2000; 43: 927-931.

[7] Greene MF. Spontaneous abortions and major malformations in women with diabetes mellitus. *Semin Reprod Endocrinol* 1999; 17: 127-136.

[8] Group GaDiFS. Multicenter survey of diabetic pregnancy in France. *Diabetes Care* 1991; 14: 994-1000.

[9] Nordstrom L, Spetz E, Wallstrom K, Walinder O. Metabolic control and pregnancy outcome among women with insulin-dependent diabetes mellitus. A twelve-year follow-up in the country of Jamtland, Sweden. *Acta Obstet Gynecol Scand* 1998; 77: 284-289.

[10] Leslie RDG, Pyke DA, John PN, White JM. Hemoglobin A1 in diabetic pregnancy. *Lancet* 1978; ii: 958-959.

[11] Miller E, Hare JW, Cloherty JP, Dunn PJ, Gleason RE, Soeldner JS, Kitzmiller JL. Elevated maternal hemoglobin A1c in early pregnancy and major congenital anomalies in infants of diabetic mothers. *N Engl J Med* 1981; 304: 1331-1334.

[12] DCCT. Pregnancy outcomes in the diabetes control and complications trial. *Am J Obstet Gynecol* 1996; 174: 1343-1353.

[13] Baynes JW, Thorpe SR. Perspectives in diabetes. Role of oxidative stress in diabetic complications. A new perspective on an old paradigm. *Diabetes* 1999; 48: 1-9.

[14] Mezzetti A, Cipollone F, Cuccurullo F. Oxidative stress and cardiovascular complications in diabetes: isoprostanes as new markers on an old paradigm. *Cardiovasc Res* 2000; 47: 475-488.

[15] Gopaul NK, Änggård EE, Mallet AI, Betteridge DJ, Wolff SP, Nourooz-Zadeh J. Plasma 8-iso-PGF2alfa levels are elevated in individuals with non-insulin dependent diabetes mellitus. *FEBS Lett* 1995; 368: 225-229.

[16] Davi G, Ciabattoni G, Consoli A, Mezzetti A, Falco A, Santarone S, Pennese E, Vitacolonna E, Bucciarelli T, Costantini F, Capani F, Patrono C. In vivo formation of 8-iso-prostaglandin f2alpha and platelet activation in diabetes mellitus: effects of improved metabolic control and vitamin E supplementation. *Circulation* 1999; 99: 224-229.

[17] Laight DW, Desai KM, Gopaul NK, Anggard EE, Carrier MJ. F2-isoprostane evidence of oxidant stress in the insulin resistant, obese Zucker rat: effects of vitamin E. *Eur J Pharmacol* 1999; 377: 89-92.

[18] Wentzel P, Welsh N, Eriksson UJ. Developmental damage, increased lipid peroxidation, diminished cyclooxygenase-2 gene expression, and lowered PGE2 levels in rat embryos exposed to a diabetic environment. *Diabetes* 1999; 48: 813-820.

[19] Gerber RT, Holemans K, O'Brien-Coker I, Mallet AI, van Bree R, Van Assche FA, Poston L. Increase of the isoprostane 8-isoprostaglandin f2alpha in maternal and fetal blood of rats with streptozotocin-induced diabetes: evidence of lipid peroxidation. *Am J Obstet Gynecol* 2000; 183: 1035-1040.

[20] Nishikawa T, Edelstein D, Du XL, Yamagishi S, Matsumura T, Kaneda Y, Yorek MA, Beebe D, Oates PJ, Hammes HP, Giardino I, Brownlee M. Normalizing mitochondrial superoxide production blocks three pathways of hyperglycaemic damage. *Nature* 2000; 404: 787-790.

[21] Greene MF, Hare JW, Cloherty JP, Benacerraf BR, Soeldner JS. First-trimester hemoglobin A1 and risk for major malformation and spontaneous abortion in diabetic pregnancy. *Teratology* 1989; 39: 225-231.

[22] Hanson U, Persson B, Thunell S. Relationship between haemoglobin A1c in early type 1 (insulin-dependent) diabetic pregnancy and the occurrence of spontaneous abortion and fetal malformation in Sweden. *Diabetologia* 1990; 33: 100-104.

[23] Combs C, Kitzmiller J. Spontaneous abortion and congenital malformations in diabetes. *Baillieres Clin Obstet Gynaecol* 1991; 5: 315-331.

[24] Rosenn B, Miodovnik M, Combs CA, Khoury J, Siddiqi TA. Glycemic thresholds for spontaneous abortion and congenital malformations in insulin-dependent diabetes mellitus. *Obstet Gynecol* 1994; 84: 515-520.

[25] Nielsen GL, Sorensen HT, Nielsen PH, Sabroe S, Olsen J. Glycosylated hemoglobin as predictor of adverse fetal outcome in type 1 diabetic pregnancies. *Acta Diabetol* 1997; 34: 217-222.

[26] Lazarow A, Kim JN, Wells LJ. Birth weight and fetal mortality in pregnant subdiabetic rats. *Diabetes* 1960; 9: 114-117.

[27] Endo A. Teratogenesis in diabetic mice treated with alloxan prior to conception. *Arch Environ Health* 1966; 12: 492-500.

[28] Brownscheidle M, Wootten V, Mathieu MH, Davis DL, Hofman IA. The effects of maternal diabetes on fetal maturation and neonatal health. *Metabolism* 1983; 32(suppl 1): 148-155.

[29] Morishima M, Ando M, Takao A. Visceroatrial heterotaxy syndrome in the NOD mouse with special reference to atrial situs. *Teratology* 1991; 44: 91-100.

[30] Horii K, Watanabe G, Ingalls TH. Experimental diabetes in pregnant mice: prevention of congenital malformations in offspring by insulin. *Diabetes* 1966; 15: 194-204.

[31] Eriksson UJ, Dahlström E, Larsson KS, Hellerström C. Increased incidence of congenital malformations in the offspring of diabetic rats and

their prevention by maternal insulin therapy. *Diabetes* 1982; 31: 1-6.

[32] Sivan E, Reece EA, Wu YK, Homko CJ, Polansky M, Borenstein M. Dietary vitamin E prophylaxis and diabetic embryopathy: morphologic and biochemical analysis. *Am J Obstet Gynecol* 1996; 175: 793-799.

[33] Viana M, Herrera E, Bonet B. Teratogenic effects of diabetes mellitus in the rat. Prevention with vitamin E. *Diabetologia* 1996; 39: 1041-1046.

[34] Simán CM, Eriksson UJ. Vitamin E decreases the occurrence of malformations in the offspring of diabetic rats. *Diabetes* 1997b; 46: 1054-1061.

[35] Simán CM, Eriksson UJ. Vitamin C supplementation of the maternal diet reduces the rate of malformation in the offspring of diabetic rats. *Diabetologia* 1997a; 40: 1416-1424.

[36] Cederberg J, Simán CM, Eriksson UJ. Combined anti-teratogenic treatment of the mother with vitamins E and C in experimental diabetic pregnancy. *Pediatr Res* 2001; in press.

[37] Wiznitzer A, Ayalon N, Hershkovitz R, Khamaisi M, Reece EA, Trischler H, Bashan N. Lipoic acid prevention of neural tube defects in offspring of rats with streptozocin-induced diabetes. *Am J Obstet Gynecol* 1999; 180: 188-193.

[38] Sakamaki H, Akazawa S, Ishibashi M, Izumino K, Takino H, Yamasaki H, Yamaguchi Y, Goto S, Urata Y, Kondo T, Nagataki S. Significance of glutathione-dependent antioxidant system in diabetes-induced embryonic malformations. *Diabetes* 1999; 48: 1138-1144.

[39] Vural P, Akgul C, Yildirim A, Canbaz M. Antioxidant defence in recurrent abortion. *Clin Chim Acta* 2000; 295: 169-177.

[40] Palmer AM, Thomas CR, Gopaul N, Dhir S, Ånggård EE, Poston L, Tribe RM. Dietary antioxidant supplementation reduces lipid peroxidation but impairs vascular function in small mesenteric arteries of the streptozotocin-diabetic rat. *Diabetologia* 1998; 41: 148-156.

[41] Sano T, Umeda F, Hashimoto T, Nawata H, Utsumi H. Oxidative stress measurements by in vivo electron spin resonance spectroscopy in rats with streptozotocin-induced diabetes. *Diabetologia* 1998; 41: 1355-1360.

[42] Lindmark D, Lindberg B, Hogstedt S. The incidence of hypertensive disease in pregnancy. *Acta Obstet Gynecol Scand Suppl* 1984; 118: 29-32.

[43] Schjetlein R, Abdelnoor M, Haugen G, Husby H, Sandset PM, Wisloff F. Hemostatic variables as independent predictors for fetal growth retardation in preeclampsia. *Acta Obstet Gynecol Scand* 1999; 78: 191-197.

[44] Davidge ST, Signorella AP, Hubel CA, Lykins DL, Roberts JM. Distinct factors in plasma of preeclamptic women increase endothelial nitric oxide or prostacyclin. *Hypertension* 1996; 28: 758-764.

[45] Buhimschi IA, Saade GR, Chwalisz K, Garfield RE. The nitric oxide pathway in pre-eclampsia: pathophysiological implications. *Hum Reprod Update* 1998; 4: 25-42.

[46] Kauma SW, Wang Y, Walsh SW. Preeclampsia is associated with decreased placental interleukin-6 production. *J Soc Gynecol Investig* 1995; 2: 614-617.

[47] Page NM, Woods RJ, Gardiner SM, Lomthaisong K, Gladwell RT, Butlin DJ, Manyonda IT, Lowry PJ. Excessive placental secretion of neurokinin B during the third trimester causes pre-eclampsia. *Nature* 2000; 405: 797-800.

[48] Adachi T, Nakabayashi M, Sakura M, Ando K. Involvement of fibrinolytic factors in mid trimester amniotic fluid with development of severe early-onset preeclampsia. *Semin Thromb Hemost* 1999; 25: 447-450.

[49] Kobayashi T, Tokunaga N, Sugimura M, Suzuki K, Kanayama N, Nishiguchi T, Terao T. Coagulation/fibrinolysis disorder in patients with severe preeclampsia. *Semin Thromb Hemost* 1999; 25: 451-454.

[50] Wetzka B, Winkler K, Kinner M, Friedrich I, Marz W, Zahradnik HP. Altered lipid metabolism in preeclampsia and HELLP syndrome: links to enhanced platelet reactivity and fetal growth. *Semin Thromb Hemost* 1999; 25: 455-462.

[51] Yamada N, Arinami T, Yamakawa-Kobayashi K, Watanabe H, Sohda S, Hamada H, Kubo T, Hamaguchi H. The 4G/5G polymorphism of the plasminogen activator inhibitor-1 gene is associated with severe preeclampsia. *J Hum Genet* 2000; 45: 138-141.

[52] Davidge ST. Oxidative stress and altered endothelial cell function in preeclampsia. *Semin Reprod Endocrinol* 1998; 16: 65-73.

[53] Zhou Y, Genbacev O, Damsky CH, Fisher SJ. Oxygen regulates human cytotrophoblast differentiation and invasion: implications for endovascular invasion in normal pregnancy and in preeclampsia. *J Reprod Immunol* 1998; 39: 197-213.

[54] DiFederico E, Genbacev O, Fisher SJ. Preeclampsia is associated with widespread apoptosis of placental cytotrophoblasts within the uterine wall. *Am J Pathol* 1999; 155: 293-301.

[55] Djurovic S, Schjetlein R, Wisloff F, Haugen G, Husby H, Berg K. Plasma concentrations of Lp(a) lipoprotein and TGF-beta1 are altered in preeclampsia. *Clin Genet* 1997; 52: 371-376.

[56] Nisell H, Erikssen C, Persson B, Carlstrom K. Is carbohydrate metabolism altered among women who have undergone a preeclamptic pregnancy? *Gynecol Obstet Invest* 1999; 48: 241-246.

[57] Walsh SW. Maternal-placental interactions of oxidative stress and antioxidants in preeclampsia. *Semin Reprod Endocrinol* 1998; 16: 93-104.

[58] Hubel CA. Oxidative stress in the pathogenesis of preeclampsia. *Proc Soc Exp Biol Med* 1999; 222: 222-235.

[59] Kabi BC, Goel N, Rao YN, Tripathy R, Tempe A, Thakur AS. Levels of erythrocyte malonyldialdehyde, vitamin E, reduced glutathione, G6PD activity and plasma urate in patients of pregnancy induced hypertension. *Indian J Med Res* 1994; 100: 23-25.

[60] Poranen A, Ekblad U, Uotila P, Ahotupa M. Lipid peroxidation and antioxidants in normal and preeclamptic pregnancies. *Placenta* 1996; 17: 401-405.

[61] Hubel CA, Kagan VE, Kisin ER, McLaughlin MK, Roberts JM. Increased ascorbate radical formation and ascorbate depletion in plasma from women with preeclampsia: implications for oxidative stress. *Free Radic Biol Med* 1997; 23: 597-609.

[62] Morris JM, Gopaul NK, Endresen MJ, Knight M, Linton EA, Dhir S, Anggard EE, Redman CW. Circulating markers of oxidative stress are raised in normal pregnancy and pre-eclampsia. *Br J Obstet Gynaecol* 1998; 105: 1195-1199.

[63] Roggensack AM, Zhang Y, Davidge ST. Evidence for peroxynitrite formation in the vasculature of women with preeclampsia. *Hypertension* 1999; 33: 83-89.

[64] Wakatsuki A, Ikenoue N, Okatani Y, Shinohara K, Fukaya T. Lipoprotein particles in preeclampsia: susceptibility to oxidative modification. *Obstet Gynecol* 2000; 96: 55-59.

[65] Walsh SW, Vaughan JE, Wang Y, Roberts LJ, 2nd. Placental isoprostane is significantly increased in preeclampsia. *FASEB J* 2000; 14: 1289-1296.

[66] Wang Y, Walsh S. Antioxidant activities and mRNA expression of superoxide dismutase, catalase, and glutathione peroxidase in normal and preeclamptic placentas. *J Soc Gynecol Investig* 1996; 3: 179-184.

[67] Poranen A, Ekblad U, Uotila P, Ahotupa M. The effect of vitamin C and E on placental lipid peroxidation and antioxidative enzymes in perfused placenta. *Acta Obstet Gynecol Scand* 1998; 77: 372-376.

[68] Wang Y, Walsh SW. Placental mitochondria as a source of oxidative stress in pre-eclampsia. *Placenta* 1998; 19: 581-586.

[69] Kossenjans W, Eis A, Sahay R, Brockman D, Myatt L. Role of peroxynitrite in altered fetal-placental vascular reactivity in diabetes or preeclampsia. *Am J Physiol Heart Circ Physiol* 2000; 278: H1311-H1319.

[70] Many A, Hubel CA, Fisher SJ, Roberts JM, Zhou Y. Invasive cytotrophoblasts manifest evidence of oxidative stress in preeclampsia. *Am J Pathol* 2000; 156: 321-331.

[71] Staff AC, Ranheim T, Henriksen T, Halvorsen B. 8-Iso-prostaglandin f(2alpha) reduces trophoblast invasion and matrix metalloproteinase activity. *Hypertension* 2000; 35: 1307-1313.

[72] Benedetto C, Valensise H, Marozio L, Giarola M, Massobrio M, Romanini C. A two-stage screening test for pregnancy-induced hypertension and preeclampsia. *Obstet Gynecol* 1998; 92: 1005-1011.

[73] Chappell LC, Seed PT, Briley AL, Kelly FJ, Lee R, Hunt BJ, Parmar K, Bewley SJ, Shennan AH, Steer PJ, Poston L. Effect of antioxidants on the occurrence of pre-eclampsia in women at increased risk: a randomized trial. *Lancet* 1999; 354: 810-816.

[74] Myatt L, Kossenjans W, Sahay R, Eis A, Brockman D. Oxidative stress causes vascular dysfunction in the placenta. *J Matern Fetal Med* 2000; 9: 79-82.

[75] Wang YP, Walsh SW, Guo JD, Zhang JY. The imbalance between thromboxane and prostacyclin in preeclampsia is associated with an imbalance between lipid peroxides and vitamin E in maternal blood. *Am J Obstet Gynecol* 1991; 165: 1695-1700.

[76] Hsu CD, Tan HY, Hong SF, Nickless NA, Copel JA. Strategies for reducing the frequency of pre-eclampsia in pregnancies with insulin-dependent diabetes mellitus. *Am J Perinatol* 1996; 13: 265-268.

[77] Hiilesmaa V, Suhonen L, Teramo K. Glycaemic control is associated with pre-eclampsia but not with pregnancy-induced hypertension in women with type I diabetes mellitus. *Diabetologia* 2000; 43: 1534-1539.

[78] Combs CA, Rosenn B, Kitzmiller JL, Khoury JC, Wheeler BC, Miodovnik M. Early-pregnancy proteinuria in diabetes related to preeclampsia. *Obstet Gynecol* 1993; 82: 802-807.

[79] Ylinen K, Raivio K, Teramo K. Haemoglobin AIc predicts the perinatal outcome in insulin-dependent diabetic pregnancies. *Br J Obstet Gynaecol* 1981; 88: 961-967.

[80] Kitzmiller J, Buchanan T, Kjos S, Combs C, Ratner R. Pre-conception care of diabetes, congenital malformations, and spontaneous abortions. *Diabetes Care* 1996; 19: 514-541.

[81] Eriksson UJ, Borg LAH, Cederberg J, Nordstrand H, Simán CM, Wentzel C, Wentzel P. Pathogenesis of diabetes-induced congenital malformations. *Ups J Med Sci* 2000; 105: 53-84.

[82] Eriksson UJ, Borg LAH. Protection by free oxygen radical scavenging enzymes against glucose-induced embryonic malformations in vitro. *Diabetologia* 1991; 34: 325-331.

[83] Eriksson UJ, Borg LAH. Diabetes and embryonic malformations. Role of substrate-induced free-oxygen radical production for dysmorphogenesis in cultured rat embryos. *Diabetes* 1993; 42: 411-419.

[84] Winn LM, Wells PG. Phenytoin-initiated DNA oxidation in murine embryo culture, and embryo-protection by the antioxidative enzymes superoxide dismutase and catalase: evidence for reactive oxygen species mediated DNA oxidation in the molecular mechanism of phenytoin teratogenicity. *Mol Pharmacol* 1995; 48: 112-120.

[85] Winn LM, Wells PG. Maternal administration of superoxide dismutase and catalase in phenytoin teratogenicity. *Free Radic Biol Med* 1999; 26: 266-274.

[86] Davis WL, Crawford LA, Cooper OJ, Farmer GR, Thomas DL, Freeman BL. Ethanol induces the generation of reactive free radicals by neural crest cells in vitro. *J Craniofac Genet Dev Biol* 1990; 10: 277-293.

[87] Kotch LE, Chen S-E, Sulik KK. Ethanol-induced teratogenesis: free radical damage as a possible mechanism. *Teratology* 1995; 52: 128-136.

[88] Chen S-Y, Sulik KK. Free radicals and ethanol-induced cytotoxicity in neural crest cells. *Alcohol Clin Exp Res* 1996; 20: 1071-1076.

[89] Muresan C, Eremia I. Ethanol stimulates the formation of free oxygen radicals in the brain of newborn rats. *Rom J Morphol Embryol* 1997; 43: 113-117.

[90] Parman T, Mahendra AS, Wiley MJ, Wells PG. Inhibition of thalidomide-initiated DNA oxidation and teratogenicity in rabbits by the free radical spin trapping agent alfa-phenyl-N-t-butylnitrone (PBN). *Fundam Appl Toxicol* 1997; 36(suppl 1): 303.

[91] Parman T, Wiley MJ, Wells PG. Free radical-mediated oxidative DNA damage in the mechanism of thalidomide teratogenicity. *Nat Med* 1999; 5: 582-585.

[92] Botto LD, Mulinare J, Erickson JD. Occurrence of congenital heart defects in relation to maternal mulitivitamin use. *Am J Epidemiol* 2000; 151: 878-884.

Chapter 5

Medical management of pregestational diabetes

Clara Lowy

Clara Lowy, MD, MSc, FRCP, Emeritus Professor of Endocrinology, Guys Kings and St. Thomas' School of Medicine.

Medical management of pregestational diabetes

Clara Lowy*

Abstract.–The team members who should be involved are identified and the importance of the principal team member, i.e., the pregnant women is stressed. Periconceptual glycaemic control is critical, as the embryo is particularly vulnerable to anamolies. Delivery of insulin and the types of insulin available together with guidelines of what constitutes adequate glycaemic control are described. The role of the serial fetal ultrasound monitoring is outlined. The importance of identifying women with microangiopathic and macroangiopathic diabetic complications is stressed and the risk to their health and their babies' health are categorised with emphasis on providing information to the women and thus allowing them to make informed choices. Glycaemic management during labour and the pros and cons of induction versus caesarean section are discussed. Insulin administration in the immediate post-partum period is outlined and the erratic glycaemic control often experienced whilst women are breast feeding is deacribed. Finally, the importance of acceptable contraception is stressed since an unplanned pregnancy tends to carry a greater risk than the risks of the different forms of contraception.

Keywords: pregestational Type I & II diabetes, pregnancy, diabetic management.

*Address for correspondence: Hospital address: Diabetic and Endocrine Day Centre, North Wing 6th Floor, St. Thomas' Hospital, London SE1 7EH, United Kingdom. Tel.: 0207 928 9292, Ext. 3791, Fax: 0207 922 8289. Home address: 44A Rosemont Road, London W3 9LY, United Kingdom. Tel.: 0208 992 2404, Fax: 0208 992 3031, E-mail: *clara.lowy@kcl.ac.uk*

General points

Diabetic pregnancy outcome has improved since the discovery and introduction of insulin 78 years ago. The perinatal mortality has decreased from 500 to less than 50 per 1000 live births and seems to be lower in countries with registers (Refs. [1–4]; Nielsen et al, 1993; von Kries et al, 1997). The factors that have contributed to this improvement are the recognition of the impotence of maternal glycaemic control, the practicality of monitoring control from preconception, the introduction of ultrasound monitoring and the expertise of the neonatologist to care for premature babies. Irrespective of the type of diabetes or complexity, there are guidelines that apply to all women [5] and these will now be described.

Registration of a pregnancy should occur at the earliest opportunity so that adjustment of diet, insulin doses and their timing can be made. Ideally staff comprising a diabetologist, obstetrician specialist diabetic nurse, midwife, dietician and paediatrician should be able to consult with the patient in a combined clinic allowing face to face communication at each antenatal visit. Frequency of visits will depend on the stage of pregnancy but usually, visits every 2 weeks are sufficient until close to term when weekly is more appropriate. What should be ascertained at the fortnightly visit? The demographic measurements of bodyweight, blood pressure, urine test for protein and ketones, random blood glucose and either fructosamine or glycated haemoglobin A1c. Ideally the biochemical measurements should be available at the consultation so that they can be discussed with the most important team member, the patient. The home blood glucose results executed between visits should be reviewed, blood glucose patterns sought and adjustments of insulin doses and diet suggested. Guidelines should be given for the timing, frequency and level of the blood glucose measurements. With the introduction of the modern pricking devices (soft click) and the simplified glucose monitors with and without memories, most women can be persuaded to carry out two preprandial and two postprandial measurements per day. There is still much discussion as to what is considered an acceptable blood glucose level but ideally they should be within the normal range. However, this results in more hypoglycaemia [6] and may also result in hypoglycaemic unawareness. Four to six mmol/l before meals and < 8 mmol/l one and half hours postprandially are a reasonable compromise. Blood glucose values should not be less than 6 mmol/l at bedtime since hypoglycaemia has been reported to occur in 75% with lower values. The numbers and timing of blood glucose measurements should be adjusted for each patient since it is easy to intimidate the women leading to falsification of results. Identification of falsified results can be detected in a number of ways; by absent finger prick marks, failure of random distribution of the terminal blood glucose figure, lack of correspondence of memory data with the women's manual recording. Direct confrontation may not solve the problem and sometimes asking the women to perform fewer tests may relieve the pressure and may result in better compliance. Routine hospitalisation to assess diabetic control is no longer necessary but may be the only way to achieve control in the few women with chaotic lifestyles. Insulin injection frequency has increased and has resulted in better glycaemic control so that most Type I diabetic women are managed with short acting/regular insulin preprandially and intermediate acting insulin at bedtime. More recently the modified insulin (lispro) with a much faster absorption profile has become popular. It has been employed in pregnancy but has been associated with development of proliferative retinopathy in 3 of 14 women [7]. Continuous subcutaneous infusion using modern adjustable pumps have gained ground in the USA but are infrequently used in the UK largely because of cost and randomised trials have shown little advantage [8]. The insulin dose increases with advancing pregnancy. During the first trimester insulin requirements depend on a number of factors. The well-controlled women with no first trimester nausea may require no change or an increase because of increased appetite. If food intake is decreased by nausea the insulin dose may fall. Typically the younger non-compliant girls whose recorded insulin dose may bear little relation to the injected dose may require much less insulin as she becomes more compliant. Once glycaemic control is satisfactory and first trimester nausea has resolved the insulin dose changes little until 22-24 weeks. Thereafter, there is a roughly 10% rise every 4 weeks with a steeper rise between 28 and 32 weeks. This is followed by a declining rise so that by 36-37 weeks insulin requirements may actually be falling, usually not associated with fetal compromise [9]. The nocturnal requirements may be especially affected. It is important for the women to record the fasting blood glucose systematically so that as the values fall she can reduce her intermediate bedtime insulin and thus avoid unpleasant nocturnal hypoglycaemic attacks. Hypoglycaemia management should be revised and glucagon kits issued to partners or other members of the household. The glycated haemoglobin or fructosamine level provides confirmation of mean blood glucose concentrations [10], but provides no data on blood glucose excursions. Uncorrected fructoasmine values fall with advancing pregnancy and HbA1c can be misleadingly low if the women has been anaemic and is responding to haematinic therapy.

Ultrasound measurements have become a valuable tool to date the pregnancy, to detect anomalies and to monitor fetal growth. Ultrasound measurements in the first trimester confirm fetal gestational age and viability. Scans at 18-22 weeks help to identify major anomalies. Special scans of the fetal heart can now identify anomalies so that either a therapeutic termination can be carried out or the neonatal team can be warned of an impending sick neonate. Serial 4-6 weekly growth scans with measurements of the biparietal diameter head and abdominal circumference and femur length provide data on satisfactory fetal growth. Despite the better glycaemic control, most units still report an excess of heavy babies [11]. Thus, a baby should be growing at least on the 50th centile especially if maternal glycaemic control is not optimal. Whilst there is no correlation between birth weight and overall glycated haemoglobin; the author has observed in his series that elevated third trimester blood glucose and HbA1c correlate with fetal abdominal circumference growth rate. Matching the fetal growth rate with the mother's glycaemic control provides some data on fetal well-being.

Management of sub-groups of diabetic women

The White classification in various versions has been used to identify degree of pregnancy risk but as duration of diabetes per se plays a much smaller part than the presence of micro- and/or macrovascular complications in predicting risk; the author has categorised risk by the latter. Thus, he will describe management based on the identified complications. The latter should have been identified at the prepregnancy visit that is covered in Dr. Steel's chapter. Type I and II diabetes are dealt in the following sections.

Management of Type I diabetes

■ With no complications

The fundi should be reviewed through dilated pupils in the second trimester. In the absence of retinopathy, hypertension and acceptable glycaemic control progression to retinopathy is absent or minimal [12]. It is worth reviewing the fundi post-partum as data has demonstrated that this is the most sensitive time for detecting retinopathy [13].

■ With microvascular complications

Retinopathy

The prevalence of retinopathy varies but as the duration of diabetes has increased from 10 to nearer 20 years in the pregnant population, the prevalence has also increased to about 30% [14]. The mechanisms causing retinopathy are still not clearly defined but increased retinal blood flow is associated with the development of retinopathy [15]. Pregnancy [16], elevated plasma glucose and hypertension all lead to increased retinal blood flow. Precipitous improvement of glycaemic control to avoid fetal anomalies may activate retinopathy. Thus, when retinopathy is present in the first trimester careful serial fundal evaluation is mandatory to assess possible progression and need for laser treatment [17]. Progression to sight-threatening retinopathy is rare but the most vulnerable women are single mothers with poor attendance records. Women who have had laser treatment for retinopathy and whose eyes are stable and who have adequate glycaemic control, seldom activate their retinopathy. They should be reviewed more frequently during the pregnancy by their attending ophthalmologist.

Nephropathy

Unlike isolated retinopathy nephropathy has major implications for both mother and fetus [18, 19]. The prevalence of proteinuria is about 5% at booking [20], but the prevalence is nearer 15% if microalbuminuria positive women are included. There are a number of aspects of renal involvement relevant to pregnancy. To conserve renal function, women with microalbuminuria are commonly treated with ACE inhibitors. Unfortunately, this class of drugs has been associated with fetal kidney anomalies and thus these drugs should be discontinued either at the prepregnancy visit or at the earliest opportunity in pregnancy [21]. If the women requires treatment for her hypertension the drugs considered safe in pregnancy are the time-honoured drugs, methyl dopa, hydralazine, and some of the beta blockers, for example labetolol. Whilst markers of diabetic nephropathy have long-term implications for the mother, they have less effect on fetal well-being unless there is an elevated plasma creatinine and concomitant hypertension and/or pre-eclampsia [20, 22]. Renal impairment, hypertension and pre-eclampsia are associated with reduced fetal growth and a possibly hypoxic fetus with a possible intrauterine death if the pregnancy is allowed to go to term. Whilst the probability of less than satisfactory fetal outcome can be related to the degree of renal complications it is impossible to predict a particular women's outcome. This is why it is so important to define and discuss all aspects of diabetic complications prepregnancy so that the women can make an informed choice. Pregnancy following renal transplantation is well described. There is, however, an approximately 10% rejection and graft loss, increased incidence of hypertension, poor fetal growth with a premature delivery of a small for dates baby. The standard immunosuppresive drugs cyclosporin, azothiaprin and steroids have not been associated with fetal anomalies and can therefore be continued throughout the pregnancy [23].

Autonomic neuropathy

Symptomatic autonomic neuropathy involving the gastrointestinal tract and/or the bladder are rare in pregnancy [24]. These women usually have had previous hospitalisation for intractable vomiting and/or recurrent urinary tract infections, and thus the clinical history will identify them. A large atonic bladder that fails to empty is often associated with a persistent infection. Not uncommonly this small group of usually non-compliant women has had past episodes of pyelonephritis and assessment of urinary tract infections throughout pregnancy is vital. Nausea with vomiting is a common complaint in the first trimester, but if due to gastric autonomic neuropathy will be more profound leading to weight loss, dehydration and decompensated diabetes. This condition should be treated as an emergency with hospitalisation, rehydration and administration of vitamin B supplements. Whilst anti-emetic medication is not ideal but is the better option if it controls the vomiting. Very occasionally parenteral nutrition may be required. Unlike the majority of diabetic women this small group will require recurrent hospitalisation.

■ With ischaemic heart disease

The vascular adaptation to pregnancy results in the cardiac output increasing by approximately 25%. This change starts to take place towards the end of the first trimester. Women with long duration of diabetes particularly if they have a history of poor glycaemic control and/or have nephropathy with hypertension are candidates for ischaemic heart disease [25]. The prepregnancy consultation should identify and evaluate these women and offer them treatment such as angioplasty or even coronary by-pass surgery, if appropriate. In the author's limited experience of two women, one with a previous infarct and the other with previous angioplasty neither had any further problems with their hearts, in three pregnancies.

Management of Type II diabetes

Type II diabetic women tend to be well into their thirties, often obese and multiparous. They are more commonly of Asian or Afro-Caribbean origin. Most are on a prescribed diet with or without a biguanide and/or a sulphonylurea. As a group they are seldom seen before the pregnancy and tend to have markedly elevated plasma glucose values. They seldom have microvascular complications since their diabetes on average is of less than 10 years duration. The challenge is to capture them before pregnancy and achieve glycaemic control. This usually means transfer to insulin. If glycaemic control is acceptable and the women is only taking a sulphonylurea, a change does need to be made as the latter have not been implicated in the development of fetal anomalies [26]. However, the sulphonylureas cross the placenta and stimulate the fetal beta cell's insulin production. For this reason, this class of drugs should be discontinued no later than the third trimester to avoid a fat hypoglycaemic neonate. NIDDM women are insulin resistant and seldom develop ketonuria, they can be managed with mixtures of short and intermediate insulin administered preprandially twice or three times a day. The Afro-Caribbean diet is qualitatively satisfactory but usually very rich in rice and carbonated sugary drinks. The Asian women tend to be thinner but also insulin resistant and easier to manage except at the time of Ramadan when timing of food intake is distorted. Although in Europe Type II diabetic women are a small percent of pregestional diabetic women, perinatal mortality is similar to the Type I diabetic women (Ref. [1]; Towner, 1995).

Management of obstetric complications

■ Pre-eclamptic toxaemia

This condition is the commonest obstetric complication and is approximately four times as common in the pregnant diabetic population compared with the background population. It can be life threatening and whilst hospital rest may allow prolongation of the pregnancy, in severe cases with accelerating hypertension, increasing proteinuria and oedema, delivery is the only option. The mechanism for the increased incidence is not known but in the Swedish survey [20], toxaemia was associated with long duration of diabetes, nephropathy, retinopathy and an elevated first trimester glycated haemoglobin.

■ Premature delivery

A premature delivery may be forced upon the mother because of worsening pre-eclampsia, poor fetal growth with concern of an impending intrauterine death or the onset of spontaneous premature labour. If the gestational age is less than 34 weeks, fetal lung maturity can be enhanced by giving the mother 12 mg of dexamethasone 12 hours apart. There is evidence that in non-diabetic pregnancies this reduces the risk of respiratory distress syndrome in the neonate. There are no adequate studies that this is beneficial in diabetic pregnancies nevertheless dexamethasone is regularly given to diabetic women. The latter is equivalent to approximately 1200 mg of hydrocortisone and makes the women very insulin resistant. Maintaining glycaemic control in order to avoid another insult to the fetus is most important. As the women are usually able to eat normally the author continues with their subcutaneous insulin doses but set up an intravenous insulin infusion and measure capillary bedside blood glucose hourly. Usually, additional intravenous insulin is not required until 4-6 hours after the first dose of dexamethasone and is required for some 12-24 hours after the second dose of dexamethasone. It was fashionable to abort premature labour by infusing a beta agonist such as Salbutamol. This causes very severe insulin resistance and also shifts potassium into cells. The combination of salbutamol infusion and dexamethsone is best avoided unless the women are managed in a high-dependency ward to avoid decompensated diabetes, ketoacidoses with fetal demise.

Management of concomitant diseases

Diabetic women have an increased incidence of other autoimmune endocrine diseases. The commonest is hypothyroidism often insidious in onset but with implications for the fetus [27]. Hormone replacement is simple but important. Hyperthyroidism has more prominent symptoms and should be treated irrespective of the diabetes. Cushing's syndrome, Addison's disease or hypopituitarism are extremely rare but the latter two can cause severe fasting hypoglycaemia. A poor appetite and falling insulin requirements should alert the clinician. Coeliac disease is associated with Type I diabetes. It is important that these women get adequate vitamin and iron supplements.

Management of labour

Despite the best efforts to normalise maternal blood glucose, about 30% of babies have a birth weight in excess of the 90th centile for gestational age [11]. The combination of a possible obstructive labour together with a failed induction has resulted in a 40-50% caesarean section rate in most units. Furthermore, the introduction of epidural anaesthesia, which effectively avoids the fetus receiving any anaesthetic and thereby abolishing the associated anaestheic neonatal pulmonary problems, has made a planned caesarean section very attractive. Caesarean sections are best carried out in the morning. Women should receive a slightly lower-intermediate insulin dose the night before. Breakfast should be substituted by a 10% dextrose intravenous infusion delivering 150 g of dextrose over 24 hours. This avoids fasting ketonaemia and excessive fluid overloading. The intravenous insulin infusion rate can be calculated by taking the total dose over the last 24 hours subtracting approximately 20-25% and dividing by 24. This, the author has found, is approximately the dose required per hour to maintain the blood glucose between 4 and 6 mmol/l. In order to fine tune the blood glucose level, bedside hourly measurements are made and a sliding scale is devised so that changes can be made for each mmol/l of change of blood glucose. Every department has their own particular regime, some will place the insulin in the dextrose solution. This has the merit of safety but provides much less flexibility. It is important to avoid both maternal hypoglycaemia and hyperglycaemia since the latter effectively stimulates fetal insulin secretion aggravating neonatal hypoglycaemia. Women who are having a planned induction need not fast until there is evidence that labour is established. The author tries to maintain flexibility by allowing a light breakfast with a slightly reduced short-acting insulin dose and then proceeding with the caesarean section protocol. Relatively few women present in labour but the same glycaemic control should be the goal.

Post-partum management including breast feeding

The increased insulin requirements of pregnancy are associated with the production of placental insulin-resistant hormones, for example, HPL, growth hormone oestrogens and progesterone. At parturition the production ceases, and as they all have short half-lives insulin sensitivity is precipitously restored. In addition if the women has laboured, the exercise may also make her more insulin sensitive. Women who have had a vaginal delivery and therefore have laboured usually require even less insulin than before pregnancy. A small dose of intermediate-acting insulin is usually sufficient. Following a caesarean section the insulin infusion rate should be halved and blood glucose maintained between 6 and 10 mmol/l. Most caesarean sections are performed under epidural anaesthesia and women are able to eat within 12 hours. Breast-feeding should be encouraged since unlike the milk formulas breast milk contains the essential long-chain fatty acids. The majority of women achieve acceptable glycaemic control with relatively few hypoglycaemic attacks in the third trimester of pregnancy, in contrast post-partum glycaemic control tends to be erratic. Breast-feeding women have been shown to require less insulin than formula-feeding women [28]. Over the first 6-8 weeks women should be advised to maintain glucose levels 2 or so mmol/l higher and not to worry about the odd value over 10 mmol/l.

Contraception

Controversy exists as to whether all modes of contraception are equally safe for diabetic as for non-diabetic women [29]. An unplanned pregnancy is the least safe option, and thus effective contraception can only be achieved with the option that is acceptable to the women.

Summary

A diabetic pregnancy still carries a 3- to 4-fold increased risk of complications for both mother and baby compared with the background population. But with adequate prepregnant glycaemic control there is less progression of the microvascular complications, a lower incidence of pre-eclampsia, the major contributers to premature delivery and excess perinatal morbidity and mortality. There is still a long way to go before the outcome of all diabetic women matches the background population.

Key points for Chapter 5 entitled Medical Management of Pregestational Diabetes

The incidence of congenital malformations of the baby of the diabetic mother has only improved marginally since Peel and Oakley reported their series in 1949.

Whilst there is a significant correlation between the first trimester HbA1c value and the incidence of malformations, it is not very dramatic. In small reported series, women who receive formal, prepregnancy counselling advice, are reported to have fewer babies with malformations. The role of a balanced diet, the addition of vitamins such as folic acid, may play an important part as glycaemic control. However, the counselled pregnant population are very much in the minority. Preparation for pregnancy remains a priority.

Perinatal mortality rates vary from country to country but even in the Scandinavian countries the baby of the diabetic mother still has a 3-4-fold higher mortality rate compared with the background population. The perinatal mortality has generally fallen over the years but the gap between the background and the diabetic population is closing all too slowly.

Prematurity is a major cause of infant mortality and morbidity, and this is largely due to the approximately doubled incidence of pre-eclamptic toxaemia in diabetic compared with non-diabetic women. The women with the poorest first trimester glycaemic control and with pregestational microalbuminuria seem to be at increased risk. Glycaemic control can be improved but microalbuminuria reflects early nephropathy. Its detection early in pregnancy can provide a warning to the caring team. Unfortunately the ACE inhibitors are contraindicated in pregnancy, as they cause fetal renal failure. Oxidative stress is increased in diabetes. However, the role of antioxidants (vitamins C and E) have not been evaluated in diabetic pregnancies.

Assessments of fetal size and gestational age optimal for delivery are still hotly debated. The majority of babies remain larger for gestational age and disproportionately fatter, and the route of delivery for a particular baby is still based on clinical habit. Most units feel comfortable with terminating the pregnancy at 38 weeks, but a primiparous women has only a 60% chance of delivering vaginally following an induction of labour. Thus, the section rate remains high (about 50%).

There are a small number of pregnancies where fetal growth is below the 50th centile and these babies have a much higher stillbirth incidence. Women with hypertension and/or renal failure are particularly at risk, also women with persistent very poor glycaemic control. Closer supervision and paradoxically an earlier delivery may offer a better chance for these infants.

There are a number of groups of women who are at additional risk. Women with preproliferative retinopathy may need laser treatment prior to a pregnancy but once their retinopathy has been stabilised they do not run additional visual risk during the pregnancy.

Women with nephropathy with plasma creatinines > 130 μmol/l at booking are at increased risk of hypertension, pre-eclamptic toxaemia and as a result of the latter a premature delivery.

Women with very long-standing Type I diabetes will have a higher incidence of coronary artery disease. Whilst myocardial infarction in pregnancy is still rare, it carries a high mortality.

The incidence of Type II diabetes is increasing and occurring at a younger age. These women are usually obese and treated with oral agents. They are not targeted and tend to present with poor glycaemic control later in pregnancy. The outcome for these pregnancies is subsequently poor. Asian and African women are particularly at risk.

The St. Vincent target of a perinatal mortality no higher than the background population is still in the far distance. Solutions depend on further understanding of the diabetic pregnancy, pathology and dedicated teamwork. This latter is graphically illustrated by the team from Estonia who presented their data to the DPSG in 2000 in Israel. Their perinatal mortality of Type I diabetic women was 290/1000 live births for 1988-93 and 63 per 1000 live births for 1994-99 following the introduction of a team approach, home glucose monitoring and appropriate insulins.

A committed team consisting of a Diabetic Physician, a Diabetic Specialist Nurse, an Obstetrician, a Midwife, a Dietician and a Neonatologist, should be available to every pregestational diabetic women.

References

[1] Connell FA, Vadheim C, Emanuel I. Diabetes in pregnancy: a population-based study of incidence, referrel for care, and perinatal mortality. *Am J Obstet Gynecol* 1985; 151: 598-603.

[2] Hanson U, Persson B. Outcome of pregnancies complicated by Type I insulin dependent diabetes in Sweden: acute pregnancy complications, neonatal mortality and morbidity. *Am J Perinatol* 1993; 10: 330-333.

[3] Casson IF, Clarke CA, Howard CV, McKendrick O, Pennycook S, Pharoa POD et al. Outcomes of pregnancy in insulin dependent diabetic women – results of a five year population cohort study. *BMJ* 1997; 315: 275-278.

[4] Hawthorne G, Robson S, Ryall EA, Roberts SH, Ward Platt MP. Prospective population based survey of outcome of pregnancy in diabetic women: results of the Northern Diabetic Pregnancy Audit 1994. *BMJ* 1997; 315: 279-281.

[5] Jardine Brown C, Dawson A, Dodds R, Gamsu H, Gillmer M, Hall M et al. Report of the pregnancy and neonatal care group. *Diabetic Med* 1996; 13: S43-S53.

[6] Rosenn BM, Miodovnik M, Holcberg G, Khoury JC, Siddiqi TA. Hypoglycemia: the price of intensive insulin therapy for pregnant women with insulin dependent diabetes mellitus. *Obstetr Gynecol* 1995; 85: 417-422.

[7] Kitzmiller JL, Main E, Ward B, Theiss T, Peterson DL. Insulin lispro and the development of proliferative diabetic retinopathy during pregnancy. *Diabetes Care* 1999; 22: 874-875.

[8] Burkart W, Hanker JP, Schneider HPG. Complications and fetal outcome in diabetic pregnancy. *Gynecol Obstet Invest* 1988; 26: 104-112.

[9] Steel JM, Johnstone FD, Hume R, Mao JH. Insulin requirements during pregnancy in women with type I diabetes. *Obstetr Gynecol* 1994; 83: 250-258.

[10] Kennedy DM, Johnson AB, Hill PG. A comparison of automated fructosamine and HbA1c methods for monitoring diabetes in pregnancy. *Ann Clin Biochem* 1998; 35: 283-289.

[11] Persson B, Hanson U. Fetal size at birth in relation to quality of blood glucose control in pregnancies complicated by pregestational diabetes mellitus. *Br J Obstetr Gynaecol* 1996; 103: 427-433.

[12] Axer-Siegel R, Hod M, Fink-Cohen S, Kramer M, Weinberger D, Schindel B, Yassur Y. Diabetic retinopathy during pregnancy. *Ophthalmology* 1996; 103: 1815-1819.

[13] Hellstedt T, Kaaja R, Teramo K, Immonen I. The effect of pregnancy on mild diabetic retinopathy. *Graefes Arch Clin Exp Ophthalmol* 1997; 235: 437-441.

[14] Reece EA, Sivan E, Francis G, Homko CJ. Pregnancy outcomes among women with and without diabetic microvascular disease (White's Classes B to FR) versus non-diabetic controls. *Am J Perinatol* 1998; 15: 549-555.

[15] Chen HC, Newsom RSB, Patel V, Cassar J, Mather H, Kohner EM. Retinal blood flow changes during pregnancy in women with diabetes. *Invest Ophthalmol Visual Sci* 1994; 35: 3199-3208.

[16] Hellstedt T, Kaaja R, Teramo K, Immonen I. Macular blood flow during pregnancy in patients with early diabetic retinopathy measured by-field entoptic simulation. *Graefes Arch Clin Exp Opthalmol* 1996; 234: 659-663.

[17] Lauszus FF, Gron PL, Klebe JG. Pregnancies complicated by diabetic proliferative retinopathy. *Acta Obstet Gynecol Scand* 1998; 77: 814-818.

[18] Kimmerle R, Zaz RP, Cupisti S, Somville T, Bender R, Pawlowski B et al. Pregnancies in women with diabetic nephropathy: long term outcome for mother and child. *Diabetologia* 1995; 38: 227-235.

[19] Kitzmiller JL, Combs CA. Diabetic nephropathy and pregnancy. *Obstetr Gynecol Clin North America* 1996; 23: 173-203.

[20] Hanson U, Persson B. Epidemiology of pregnancy-induced hypertension and preeclampsia in Type I (insulin dependent) diabetic pregnancies in Sweden. *Acta Obstet Gynecol Scand* 1998; 77: 620-624.

[21] Hanssen M, Keirse MJNC, Vankelecom F, Van Assche FA. Fetal and neonatal effects of treatment with angiotensin-converting enzyme inhibitors in pregnancy. *Obstet Gynecol* 1991; 78: 128-135.

[22] Gordon M, Landon MB, Samuels P, Hissrich S, Gabbe SG. Perinatal outcome and long term follow-up associated with modern management of diabetic nephropathy. *Obstet Gynecol* 1996; 87: 401-409.

[23] Armenti VT, Ahlswede KM, Ahlswede BA, Jarrell BE, Moritz MJ, Burke JF. National transplantation pregnancy registry-outcomes of 154 prgnancies in cyclosporine-treated female kidney transplant recipients. *Transplantation* 1994; 57: 502-506.

[24] Macleod AF, Smith SA, Sonksen PH, Lowy C. The problem of autonomic neuropathy in diabetic pregnancy. *Diabetic Med* 1990; 7: 80-82.

[25] Bagg W, Henley PG, Macpherson P, Cundy TF. Pregnancy in women with diabetes and ischaemic

heart disease. *Aust NZ J Obstet Gynecol* 1999; 39: 99-102.

[26] Towner D, Kjos SL, Leung B, Montoro MM, Xiang A, Mestman JH et al. Congenital malformations in pegnancies complicated by NIDDM. *Diabetes Care* 1995; 18: 1446-1451.

[27] Bech K, Hoier-Madsen M, Feldt-Rasmussen U, Jensen BM, Molsted-Pedersen L, Kuhl C. Thyroid function and autoimmune manifestations in insulin-dependent diabetic mellitus during and after pergnancy. *Acta Endocrinologica (Copenh)* 1991; 124: 534-539.

[28] Alban Davies H, Clark JDA, Dalton KJ, Edwards OM. Insulin requirements of diabetic women who breast feed. *BMJ* 1989; 289: 1357-1358.

[29] Skouby SO, Molsted-Pedersen L, Petersen KR. Contraception for women with diabetes: an update. *Baillieres Clin Obstetr Gynecol* 1991; 5(2): 493-503.

[30] Nielsen GL, Nielsen PH. Outcome of 328 pregnancies in 205 women with insulin-dependent diabetes mellitus in the County of Northern Jutland from 1976 to 1990. *Eur J Obstetr Reprod Biol* 1993; 50: 33-38.

[31] von Kries R, Kimmerle R, Schmitd JE, Hachmeister A, Bohm O, Wolf HG. Pregnancy outcomes in mothers with pregestational diabetes: a population-based study in North Rhine (Germany) from 1988 to 1993. *Eur J Pediatr* 1997; 156: 963-967.

Chapter 6

Care of the pregnant diabetic woman

L. Cabero-Roura, Ma. José Cerqueira

L. Cabero-Roura
Ma. José Cerqueira
Hospital Valle Hebron, Passeig Vall Hebron 119, Barcelona, 08035, Spain.

Chapter 6

Care of the pregnant diabetic woman

Care of the pregnant diabetic woman

L. Cabero-Roura*, Ma. José Cerqueira

Abstract.—The main goal of pregnancy follow up in the diabetic patient is to keep carbohydrate metabolism under normal limits, since this is the best approach to prevent fetal consequences of hyperglycemia, such as malformations, growth and development disturbances, placental restriction and neonatal morbidity. A pre-conceptional investigation is warranted to evaluate the status of the diabetic patient, including assessment of chronic complications and timely treatment where indicated, and to establish the existence of contraindications to pregnancy. During pregnancy, a strict control of glucose levels is essential to ensure fetal wellbeing and appropriate growth. Recommendations for nutritional and insulin regimes are discussed in this review. Labour and delivery of the diabetic mother should be conducted according to routine protocols, although the rate of caesarean section in type I diabetic patients is higher than in non-diabetic women. Strict glycemic control during labor is essential in insulin-dependent patients to prevent neonatal hypoglycaemia. For the diabetic pregnant patient, whether previous or developing during pregnancy, the puerperium is the time to plan the future.

Keywords: diabetes, macrosomia, hypoglycemy, hidramnios, gestational diabetes, pregestational diabetes.

*Address for correspondence: L. Cabero-Roura, Hospital Valle Hebron, Passeig Vall Hebron 119, Barcelona, 08035, Spain. E-mail: lcaberor@meditex.es.

Pregestational clinical practice

The complications of diabetes in pregnancy are related to a greater or lesser extent to the degree of metabolic control in the pregnant woman. Early complications, abortions and foetal malformations are determined by the blood glucose levels at the time of conception and, as such, can only be prevented if pregnancy begins in a situation of euglycaemia, or as near to that situation as possible. It is from this concept that pregestational clinical practice is derived, the objectives of which are: (a) to evaluate the stage of development of the diabetes, to identify chronic complications, to treat them if necessary and to analyse possible contra-indications to the pregnancy; (b) to detect any cause of sterility or infertility, as well as potential risks unrelated to the diabetes; (c) to establish an effective contraceptive method until an adequate blood glucose profile is obtained; (d) to obtain the maximum co-operation of the patient and their partner, improving their level of information and training from both a metabolic and an obstetric viewpoint, according to the extent of their previous diabetological education; (e) to adjust the number of daily blood glucose tests and the dietary and insulin treatment to obtain adequate glucose levels so as to allow pregnancy. In patients with severe nephropathy or coronary heart disease, pregnancy should not be recommended as the prognosis for it is poor and life expectancy may be reduced. If there are proliferative or preproliferative retinal lesions, this is the time for their photocoagulation.

Various authors have shown a reduction in the rate of congenital malformations in those patients who have followed a programme of intensive preconception treatment compared to those who embarked on pregnancy without any monitoring. Fuhrmann observed an incidence of malformations of 0.8% in the first group as opposed to 7.5% in the second in a multicentre, prospective Diabetes in Early Pregnancy Study which found figures of 4.9 and 9%, respectively [1, 2]. Although it is recommended that all women with DMID and DMNID should attend preconception clinics, the degree of care given to them is still disproportionately low, partly because of the lack of information of the patients and partly because of their resistance to or abandonment of the strict protocol that is proposed to them. Those women treated with oral antidiabetics have to replace them with insulin during this period because their safety during pregnancy is uncertain. Second-generation hypoglycaemic agents which do not cross the placental barrier have been suggested in the treatment of non-insulin-dependent gestational diabetics. However, it should be borne in mind that blood glucose profiles are usually not normalized to the same degree as with insulin.

Prenatal diagnosis

The basic aim is the diagnosis of congenital malformations. Diabetes is not related to an increase in the number of chromosomal abnormalities; therefore invasive techniques such as amniocentesis and chorionic villus biopsy are not indicated in these patients unless they have risk factors other than diabetes, such as advanced age, previous family history, etc. The determination of B-HCG and α-foetoprotein in the serum of pregnant women is of less value than in non-diabetic pregnancies. α-Foetoprotein values in maternal serum indicative of a defect of the neural tube are lower than usual, require correction and their usefulness is disputed. HCG levels are also reduced, although without significant differences and a correction factor does not need to be used [3].

The ultrasound examination performed at about 20 weeks of pregnancy is the best method of screening for malformations in CDM. Defects of the neural tube are those identified with greatest accuracy, with results of up to 100% being quoted [4]. At the other end of the spectrum are cardiac malformations. Generally the most severe are identified in the second trimester, but the mild forms pass unnoticed [5].

Maternofoetal metabolic control

■ Metabolic control

As early as 1928, Dr. White advised that excellent control of blood glucose levels was essential for foetal well-being and suggested that hyperglycaemia in the placental blood was possibly related to excessive foetal growth [6].

In 1972, Karlsson and Kjellmer demonstrated the relationship existing between maternal blood sugar levels and perinatal mortality [7], and in a review of the literature conducted in 1980 by Jovanovic and Peterson a linear correlation was observed over the years between the two [8].

Glucose levels change during pregnancy due to the progressive increase in the anti-insulin hormones. Daily monitoring of blood glucose levels is therefore essential. The determination of glycosylated proteins (Hb, fructosamine, albumin, etc.) is useful in establishing the mean glucose levels during the previous weeks and in this sense they are generic indicators of the good or poor global metabolic control that has been achieved. However, the information which they provide is late in being obtained and clinical decisions cannot be based on them. The number of daily measurements of capillary blood glucose and the time at which these measurements are performed vary according to the centre, although in general at least four are recommended daily. Whereas in pregestational diabetics the preprandial blood glucose levels need to be known in order to calculate the doses of insulin required, in gestational diabetics it appears more useful to determine postprandial glucose levels since these have the best relationship to the subsequent appearance of macrosomia. Ketonuria should also be determined, especially in the first hour of the morning, since it is during the night that the pregnant woman has a greater tendency to exhibit fasting hypoglycaemia.

■ Diet

This is a question that is subject to periodic discussion. After many years of using low-calorie diets, the American Diabetes Association (ADA) in 1979 recommended a normal-calorie diet comprising 20% proteins, less than 30% fats and 50-60% carbohydrates (CH), restricting cholesterol and saturated fatty acids and increasing fibre, thus delaying gastric emptying and intestinal absorption. In the most recent recommendations, a percentage of 10-20% proteins is still included, with the remainder being distributed between fats and carbohydrates so that there is less than 10% saturated fatty acids and no more than 10% polyunsaturated fatty acids, 60-70% of the calories being assigned to monosaturated fatty acids and carbohydrates [9]. The diet must be divided over the day in such a way that hyperglycaemic peaks and prolonged periods of fasting are avoided. In general, six daily meals are proposed, the three main ones plus three supplementary ones in mid-morning, mid-afternoon (tea) and before retiring, with the intention of avoiding nocturnal hypoglycaemia.

An appropriate diet in obese women is a controversial subject. In general, it is accepted that pregnancy is not the right time to lose weight. Therefore, very restrictive diets which cause ketonuria are not recommended as long as moderate restrictions are observed. Ketonuria has been associated with a reduction in the intellectual coefficient of neonates, although not all authors have confirmed the relationship. Peterson and Jovanovic recommend a calorie intake in gestational diabetics of 30 kcal/kg of actual weight for pregnant women of normal weight, 35-40 for women of low weight, 24 for moderately obese women (120-150% of the ideal weight) and 12 for severely obese women (more than 150% of the ideal weight) with a proportion of 20% proteins, 40% fats and 40% CH, because they observed that the postprandial glucose peak corresponded exactly to the quantity of carbohydrates present in the food [10]. Although fibre-rich diets reduce postprandial blood glucose levels and insulin requirements in non-pregnant diabetics, the results in pregnant women have not been so satisfactory. Ney observed a reduction in the insulin requirements using fibre-rich diets, but no lower postprandial blood glucose levels [11] and Reece, in a randomised study in which he compared a fibre-rich diet with that recommended by the ADA, was unable to demonstrate either of the two points, although he observed a smaller number of episodes of hypoglycaemia with fewer glycaemic excursions in pregnant women receiving the fibre-rich diet [12].

■ Insulin

Insulin must be used during pregnancy in all DMID and in DMNID and GD if the defined metabolic objectives cannot be obtained by diet, or by diet and exercise. During pregnancy, insulin requirements alter rapidly. The insulin regimens and the doses vary with the type of diabetes and individual requirements, and also with the centre. It may be stated that there is no single correct regimen, but various combinations of insulin, diet and exercise may be appropriate if they maintain normoglycaemia. In type 1 DM, the most common regimen involves the use of multiple doses of insulin: one or more doses of intermediate-acting insulin to maintain suitable preprandial blood glucose levels and normal insulin at each of the principal meals to prevent postprandial hyperglycaemia. The average requirements are 0.86 IU/kg in the first trimester, 0.95 IU/kg in the second and 1.2 IU/kg in the third [13]. Continuous administration of subcutaneous insulin by means of an infusion pump has theoretical advantages over the injection of repeated doses because it simulates physiological secretion better. However, no differences have been found between the two forms of insulinisation in terms of the quality of the blood glucose control achieved [14]. On the other hand, although they are generally safe, there have been descriptions of complications which may be particularly serious in pregnancy, such as severe hypoglycaemia, ketoacidosis or cutaneous abscesses. Its use is limited in pregnant women and generally confined to very labile patients in whom acceptable blood glucose profiles cannot be maintained with the multiple-dose programme.

In gestational diabetics, it is recommended that the administration of insulin is instituted when preprandial blood glucose levels exceed 105 mg/dl or postprandial blood glucose levels are greater than 140 mg/dl 1 hour after food or 120 mg/dl after 2 hours, although the disparity in the criteria in this case is very marked. The loading dose is 0.2 IU of insulin NPH per kg of bodyweight in a single daily injection administered in the morning or before retiring to bed (depending on the time of day at which peak glucose levels are observed). The percentage insulinisation in gestational diabetics varies substantially. In our centre the average figures are 30%.

Foetal monitoring of children of diabetic mothers

■ Monitoring of foetal growth

Macrosomia is the most obvious manifestation of diabetic foetopathy in the intra-uterine stage. The best option currently available to us is to undertake systematic ultrasound scans, although these have a high margin of error.

Macrosomal children of diabetic mothers have a disproportionate growth with a high weight/height quotient. The cranial circumference is normal, but there is an increase in the shoulders and trunk relative to the head. A large number of references have been found in the literature that attempt to evaluate the predictive capacity of various ultrasonographic parameters, abdominal measurements being possibly the most reliable for detecting macrosomia. Using only the abdominal circumference (AC) and undertaking ultrasonography in the 7 days before parturition, Tamura found a positive predictive value (PV+) of 78% and a negative value (PV−) of 81% if the AC was above the 90th percentile [15]. With figures of AC >36 cm and an ultrasound/parturition interval of 2 days, Pedersen reported a PV+ of 80% and a PV− of 91% [16]. Serial ultrasound scans can detect the onset of acceleration of growth in CDM. The AC is the most sensitive biometric parameter under our criterion, its growth being preceded in 30% of cases by a slight increase in amniotic fluid.

With the aim of increasing the predictability of ultrasonographic measurements, a large number of mathematical formulae have been developed which claim to calculate foetal weight. Some authors consider that the estimation of foetal weight is more sensitive than biometric parameters in detecting macrosomia. Levine, using Hadlock's curve, obtained sensitivity, specificity and PV+ of 50, 90 and 52%, respectively. In addition, false positive ultrasound scans affect the obstetric treatment of these patients because those in whom macrosomia was diagnosed were also diagnosed as having a larger number of abnormalities during parturition and had a greater percentage of caesarean sections, although in fact the neonate's weight was normal [17].

Berstein has proposed using different parameters to evaluate the impairment of CDM. Given that one of the characteristics of these foetuses is the accumulation of fatty tissue, particularly subcutaneously, the ultrasonographic identification of this would enable a diabetic foetopathy to be detected before above-normal growth occurred [18].

However, the determination of foetal size ultimately does not offer precise information about the degree of impairment. A number of factors intervene in the final weight of a neonate, it being very difficult, not to mention impossible, to determine in each case what contribution each of them has made. On the other hand, the growth of the CDM is dysharmonious and affects some tissues more than others, particularly fatty tissue. In this sense it would be more correct to evaluate the "degree of foetopathy" expressed by the level of foetal hyperinsulinaemia, which is the cause of the problem, rather than evaluating the degree of macrosomia which is no more than one of its manifestations. This idea was the starting point for the attempts to use insulin or peptide C levels in the amniotic fluid as indicators of foetal hyperinsulinism which, although used commonly by some groups, are of disputed clinical use.

■ Monitoring of foetal well-being

As the time at which diabetic pregnancies are ended has been extended, so the morbidity and mortality due to prematurity has decreased substantially. However, the prolongation of the period spent by the foetus in utero requires the availability of a suitable method for determining their state of well-being to detect any potential state of distress before it becomes irreversible. Despite this, there is no agreement about what type of tests of well-being should be performed on diabetic patients, with what frequency and from what time, with the existence of such disparate criteria as the performance of periodic tests from a specific week of pregnancy, limiting the tests in pregestational diabetics to those with poor metabolic control, or not performing systematic tests in gestational diabetics.

The *biochemical methods* which aroused such hopes during the 1970s are now obsolete. The monitoring of *foetal movements* (FM) by the mother is the simplest and oldest method of monitoring foetal well-being, although it has a considerable percentage of error. False negatives (identification of false FM) are fairly low, less than 1%, but false positives may be as high as 60%. In fact, when tested under ultrasonographic control in the third trimester of pregnancy, only a third of foetal movements are perceived by the mother. It is assumed that when the number of movements decreases the foetus may be in a poor condition because a reduction in activity has been observed prior to intra-uterine death, but it has not been possible to establish specific patterns of normality. Mulder studied body and breathing movements in near-term foetuses of diabetic mothers but found no difference in the method of moving from that in the normal population [19]. Sadovsky obtained the same results in the last 2 months of pregnancy, although between weeks 25 and 32 he reported less motility than in non-diabetic patients. Hypoglycaemia in diabetic women is conventionally associated with a reduction in foetal activity, but increased activity has also been observed [20].

The *continuous registration of FHR* before parturition has represented one of the most important advances in the control of foetal well-being. In fact, since its introduction into clinical practice, the other methods have been relegated to second place. On the basis of numerous studies, it has been possible to establish a relationship between certain manifestations of FHR and the degree of foetal well-being. This relationship, even though it is increasingly strict, is not however desirable, particularly in terms of levels of foetal health or long-term prognosis. The non-stress test (NST) has been rapidly popularised as the primary method of evaluation because of its non-invasiveness, simplicity, rapidity, ease of interpretation and cheapness. However, questions such as the criteria of interpretation, sensitivity, specificity, reproducibility, predictive value and prognostic significance of atypical patterns are the subject of dispute. There is no unanimity either about the criteria of use and the predictive value of FHR tests in diabetic pregnancies. The possible occurrence of unforeseen situations, such as hypoglycaemia, ketosis, etc., undermines the prognostic value since it is difficult to calculate for what length of time the foetus may be considered to be in a good condition after a satisfactory test is obtained. In a group of 426 diabetics in whom a NST was performed weekly, Barret found six antepartum deaths, a higher figure than that expected in other risk situations [21]. Miller observed three intra-uterine deaths in 48 pregnant women with DMID between 4 and 7 days after presenting a reactive NST [22]. Dicker suggested that the changes in characteristics of activity described in normal foetuses do not develop at the same gestational age in the foetuses of a diabetic mother, possibly because of a lack of cerebral maturation, which tends more to suggest a problem of interpretation of the NST in this group [23]. In the stress test (ST) also there is no uniformity in terms of its practice and evaluation; however, the prognostic power of a negative test is high. In various studies inolving a total of 493 insulin-dependent diabetics, it has been found that no foetal deaths occurred in metabolically stable patients in the week following a negative test [24].

The *biophysical profile* described by Maning attempts to improve on the predictive value of the FHR test by introducing other parameters such as foetal movements, breathing movements, tone and reactivity of the foetus. Few studies have evaluated the biophysical profile in diabetic patients. Golde observed that, determined after a reactive NST, the biophysical profile does not appear to provide additional information about the state of the foetus. Conversely, after a non-reactive NST, scores of more than eight are associated with a high probability that the foetus will be in a good state. However, although a high number of profiles were performed in the first group, the second was very reduced [25]. Johnson observed a good relationship between the score obtained on the biophysical profile and neonatal morbidity, but was unable to demonstrate the superiority of the profile over NST [26]. There is little experience in diabetic women with the use of the *acoustic stimulation test*, although there are doubts as to its safety and recently the risk of inducing intense foetal bradycardia has been reported. The study of the resistance to blood flow in various maternal and foetal vessels by means of *Doppler velocimetry* yields information about the state of the foetus and the difficulties of interchange at the placental level, although the results obtained are sometimes contradictory. Bracero found a relationship between the Doppler values in the third trimester of pregnancy and blood glucose levels measured sporadically in diabetic patients [27]. Carrera reported changes in flow in the umbilical and arcuate artery in diabetic patients compared with normal pregnant women; however, he was unable to establish a linear correlation between the Doppler values and those of maternal blood glucose [28]. Dicker observed an altered S/D ratio only in diabetics with vasculopathy, but found no connection between mean glucose or HbA_{1c} levels and the S/D ratio [29]. Iswhimatzu for his part found no relationship between the ratio obtained from the Doppler and plasma fructosamine or glucose, unless it exceeded 300 mg/dl, in which case a transient change was produced [30].

■ Monitoring of foetal pulmonary maturity

The incidence of hyaline membrane has declined dramatically in diabetic pregnant women, to a large extent because prematurity in these patients has been reduced and to a large extent also because better metabolic control has attenuated the deleterious effects of insulin on the foetal lung. At the same time, studies of pulmonary maturity by evaluating phospholipids in the amniotic fluid have been losing ground. Elective induction prior to term is becoming increasingly unusual and the concern about obtaining an immature foetus is less. Although the usefulness of the lecithin/sphingomyelin ratio in pregnant diabetic women has been questioned and it has been proposed that higher figures than those accepted by the non-diabetic population should be considered normal, in many series a low incidence of respiratory distress has been observed with ratios greater than 2.0. Cabero analysed the palmitic acid values and the palmitic/stearic ratio in diabetic patients and found no differences between these and the control group. Likewise, the predictive value of palmitic acid in terms of pulmonary maturity was similar in the two groups [31].

Parturition and puerperium

■ Termination of pregnancy

The approach to the time at which the diabetic pregnancy is terminated has altered substantially with the improvement in the control of patients during pregnancy. At present, the better understanding of the causes of intra-uterine death enables the pregnancy to be maintained for longer as a result of the ability to manipulate them and to minimise their effect. Under our criterion, pregnant diabetic women should begin parturition spontaneously and pregestational diabetics should go as near to term as possible, assuming that the foetal and maternal condition permits. Probably the approach to pregnant diabetic women is one of the most disputed points, since there are authors who support induction at term if the foetus is macrosomal. We do not adopt this criterion, except when we find active growth, so that in our environment, and contrary to what other results may suggest, the probability of delivery by caesarean section is greater in the case of induction than of suspected ultrasonographic macrosomia with the institution of spontaneous parturition. On the other hand, the majority of weights are normal in our population and the rates of macrosomia are low, both in the non-diabetic population (3.7%) and in gestational (4.6%) or pregestational diabetics (12.1%). Weights equal to or greater than 4500 g only account for 0.5%, without there being any significant difference in diabetic pregnant women.

However, there are still situations in which non-spontaneous delivery, whether preterm or otherwise, is the only solution to obtain a good result. The decision for termination may be taken in three circumstances: (a) when the cause is acute and the situation serious, so that it is not possible to defer extraction without risk of foetal death or severe maternal injury (suspected foetal distress, eclampsia, etc.). (b) As a prophylactic measure to avoid the occurrence of problems in cases of poor development (poor maternal metabolic compensation, progressive macrosomia, mild preeclampsia, delayed growth, etc.). (c) For circumstances extraneous to the process (previous caesarean section, maternal psychological stress because of the failure of previous pregnancies, etc.). In these cases the pregnancy should not be ended before week 38 or without a previous examination providing information about adequate foetal pulmonary maturity.

■ Care at parturition

From an obstetrical viewpoint, parturition in the diabetic patient should not differ from that of a pregnant woman without a metabolic disorder. The route of delivery chosen, the techniques of cervical ripening or induction, should be the same in both cases. However, the incidence of caesarean section is higher, particularly in pregestational diabetics, with figures of more than 50 and up to 75% being reported. This high prevalence is due both to a more permissive approach at the time of deciding on intervention and a greater number of foetal (foetopelvic disproportion, fear of shoulder dystocia in macrosomia, foetal distress, etc.), or maternal indications (failed induction, poor obstetrical conditions, etc.). Reducing the incidence, although this is a common aim, is not as simple as it might appear. Delay at the time of induction in insulin-dependent diabetics may not only reduce the number of caesarean sections, but may increase the percentage of macrosomias and shoulder dystocias. In our environment (3550 parturitions/year, 0.6% pregestational diabetics and 8.5% gestational diabetics) the number of caesarean sections is also greater in the latter. The percentage of caesarean sections is 15.2% overall in non-diabetics and 20% in diabetics, increasing to 36% in pregestational diabetics. Elective caesarean sections represent 3.1% of the normal population and 8% in diabetics and there are also more inductions in the latter (12.5% vs. 7.4%).

Intrapartum metabolic control is of particular importance, both for the mothers in the case of DMID and for the foetuses in any case. The incidence of neonatal hypoglycaemia, for example, is associated with high maternal blood glucose levels during parturition. Strict monitoring of foetal well-being is required with continuous monitoring of the heart rate to detect any early signs of distress, which may be more acute in CDM. The administration of high doses of glucose during parturition has been associated with foetal acidosis in both diabetic and non-diabetic women. The objective is to keep the mother normoglycaemic, between 70 and 90 mg/dl, which is achieved with an adequate intravenous provision of glucose and low insulin doses. In order to ensure that maternal blood glucose levels remain stable and to adjust the precise doses of insulin, hourly capillary blood glucose tests must be performed throughout parturition. If foetal distress is detected and treated with β-mimetics, the doses of insulin must be doubled compared to those administered previously and the capillary blood glucose test repeated at 30 minutes. If it is decided to perform an elective caesarean, it should be scheduled for the first hour of the morning because the patient will still have the beneficial effects of the intermediate-acting insulin administered the previous night and it will not be necessary to add glucose supplements or insulin before the foetal extraction.

■ Care in the puerperium

After parturition, the insulin requirements fall abruptly with the disappearance of the placenta and as the hormones which act as hyperglycaemic agents decrease.

At the same time the sensitivity to insulin increases and there is a tendency for repeated episodes of hyperglycaemia. On the other hand, it is not essential for the blood glucose levels to remain within such strict limits as during pregnancy since the insulin regimens and doses may be simplified. However, there is no agreement as to which are the most suitable, both continuous intravenous administration and intermittent subcutaneous administration being proposed. Different methods may encourage the adaptation of the doses of insulin, such as suppressing them after parturition and reinstating them when baseline blood glucose levels exceed 110 mg/dl or when the levels exceed 160 mg/dl 1 hour postprandially, or reducing them to half the previous dose in the case of vaginal deliveries and a third in caesarean sections on reinstation of administration.

Years ago the ability of diabetic patients to breast feed was called into question. The high percentage of premature births, complications during labour, poor neonatal development and severe metabolic abnormalities interfered in the process. However, at present, if in general a good degree of metabolic control is obtained and parturition occurs at term, there does not appear to be any reason why diabetics who so wish should not breast feed their children. The episodes of hypoglycaemia that are frequent in these patients, particularly in the first week postpartum and immediately after breast feeding, may have a negative effect. Hypoglycaemia may reduce the blood flow to the gland and the secretion of lactose [32]. However, in patients with good metabolic control there do not appear to be variations in the volume of composition of the milk, except for a very high glucose content. Breast feeding should be actively advocated in diabetic patients, not only because of the advantages which it offers to the general population (composition, transmission of immunoglobulins, etc.), but because it may also have a protective effect against the onset of type 2 diabetes. In addition, there is added value in the immediate puerperium since the early institution of maternal lactation reduces neonatal hypoglycaemia, which occurs in our population in less than 15% of pregestational and 4% of gestational diabetics.

In both types of patients, those with gestational and pregestational diabetes, the puerperium is the time for planning future strategies. In pregestational diabetics, on the one hand, the strictness of the treatment that will be followed should be taken into consideration, evaluating the cost/benefit of using a more or less intensive regimen in the medium and long term. On the other hand, the partner's desire for children should also be considered, making them aware of the need to plan the next pregnancy at the most appropriate time and establishing the most suitable contraceptive method in each case. Gestational diabetics must undergo a 2-hour OGTT (extractions at 0, 30, 60 and 120 minutes) with 75 g of glucose in order to be reclassified definitively. The blood glucose curve may be established at the first postpartum visit or 6 weeks after parturition or the suppression of lactation when all the hormonal stimuli have disappeared. Patients with gestational diabetes have a greater risk of the disorder recurring in subsequent pregnancies and developing diabetes in the future. O'Sullivan found an incidence of diabetes of 50.4% at 20 years [33], while other authors report very high percentages within shorter periods of time. In our population we observe 4% diabetes at the first postpartum OGTT and 26% abnormal curves in the follow-up after one year.

References

[1] Fuhrmann K, Risker H, Semmler K et al. Prevention of congenital malformations in infants of insulin-dependent diabetic mothers. *Diabetes Care* 1983; 6: 219.

[2] Mills JL, Knopp RH, Simpson JL et al. The NICHD-Diabetes in Early Pregnancy Study: lack of relation of increased malformation rates in infants of diabetic mothers to glycemic control during organogenesis. *N Engl J Med* 1988; 318: 671.

[3] Wald NG, Cuckle HS, Densem JW, Stone RW. Maternal serum unconjugated oestriol and chorionic gonadotrophin in pregnancies with insulin-dependent diabetes: implications for Down's syndrome screening. *Br J Obstet Gynecol* 1992; 99: 51.

[4] Hashimoto BE, Mahoney BS, Filly RA et al. Sonography, a complementary examination to alpha-fetoprotein testing for fetal neural tube defects. *J Ultrasound Med* 1985; 4: 307.

[5] Greene MF, Benacerraf BR. Prenatal diagnosis in diabetic gravidas: utility of ultrasound and maternal serum alpha-fetoprotein screening. *Obstet Gynecol* 1991; 77: 520.

[6] White P. Diabetes in pregnancy. In: Joslin EP, Ed. The treatment of diabetes mellitus, edition 4. Philadelphia: Lea & Febiger, 1928: 870–872.

[7] Karlsson K, Kjellmer I. The outcome of diabetic pregnancies in relation to the mother's blood sugar level. *Am J Obstet Gynecol* 1972; 112: 213.

[8] Jovanovic L, Peterson CM. Management of the pregnant, insulin-dependent diabetic woman. *Diabetes Care* 1980; 3: 63.

[9] American Diabetes Association. Nutrition recommendations and principles for people with diabetes mellitus. *Diabetes Care* 2000; 21(suppl 1).

[10] Peterson CM, Jovanovic-Peterson L. Percent carbohydrate and glycemic response to breakfast, lunch and dinner in women with gestational diabetes. *Diabetes* 1991; 40(suppl 2): 172.

[11] Ney D, Hollingsworth DR, Cousin L. Decreased insulin requirement and improved control of diabetes in pregnant women given a high-carbohydrate, high-fiber, low-fat diet. *Diabetes Care* 1982; 5(5): 529.

[12] Reece EA, Hagay Z, Gay Ll, et al. A randomized clinical trial of a fiber enriched diabetic diet versus the standard American Diabetes Association recommended diet in the management of diabetes mellitus in pregnancy.

[13] Langer O. Maternal glycemic criteria for insulin therapy in gestational diabetes mellitus. *Diabetes Care* 1998; 21(1): B91–B98.

[14] Coustan.

[15] Tamura RK, Sabbagha RE, Depp R et al. Diabetic macrosomia: accuracy of third trimester ultrasound. *Obstet Gynecol* 1986; 67: 828.

[16] Pedersen JF, Molsted-Pedersen L. Sonographic estimation of fetal weight in diabetic pregnancy. *Br J Obstet Gynecol* 1992; 99: 475.

[17] Levine AB, Lockwood CJ, Brown B et al. Sonographic diagnosis of the large for gestational age fetus at term: Does it make a difference? *Obstet Gynecol* 1992; 79: 55.

[18] Berstein IM, Catalano PM. Ultrasonographic estimation of fetal body composition for children of diabetic mother. *Radiology* 1991; 26: 722.

[19] Mulder EJ, O'Brien MJ, Levis YL et al. Body and breathing movements in near-term fetuses and newborn infants. *Early Hum Dev* 1990; 24: 131.

[20] Hoelden KP, Jovanovic L et al. Increased fetal activity with low maternal blood glucose levels in pregnancies complicated by diabetes. *Am J Perinatol* 1984; 1: 161.

[21] Barrett JM, Salyer SL et al. The non-stress test: an evaluation of 1000 patients. *Am J Obstet Gynecol* 1981; 141: 153.

[22] Miller JM, Horger EO. Antepartum heart rate testing in diabetic pregnancy. *J Reprod Med* 1985; 30: 515.

[23] Dierker LJ, Pillay S, Sorokin Y, Rosen MG. The change in fetal activity periods in diabetic and non diabetic pregnancies. *Am J Obstet Gynecol* 1982; 143: 181.

[24] Landon MB, Gabbe SG. Antepartum fetal surveillance in gestational diabetes mellitus. *Diabetes* 1985; 34: 50.

[25] Golde SH, Montoro M, Good-Anderson B et al. The role of nonstress test, fetal biophysical profile, and contraction stress in an outpatient management of insulin requiring diabetic pregnancies. *Am J Obstet Gynecol* 1984; 148: 269.

[26] Johnson JM, Lange IR, Harman CR et al. Biophysical profile scoring in the management of the diabetic pregnancy. *Obstet Gynecol* 1988; 72: 841.

[27] Bracero L, Schulmann H, Fleicher A et al. Umbilical artery velocimetry in diabetes and pregnancy. *Obstet Gynecol* 1986; 68: 654.

[28] Carrera JM, Izquierdo M, Alegre M, y cols. Fluxometria Doppler en la gestación asociada a diabetes. En: Cabero L, Leiva A, Eds. Diabetes y Embarazo. Clinica Ginecológica 12/3. Barcelona: Salvat Editores, 1989: 221-229.

[29] Dicker D, Goldman JA, Yosahaya A. Umbilical artery velocimetry insulin dependent diabetes mellitus pregnancies. *J Perinatol Med* 1990; 18: 391.

[30] Ishimatsu J, Joshimura C, Nanabe A et al. Umbilical artery blood flow velocity waveforms in pregnancies complicated by diabetes mellitus. *Arcg Gynecol Obstet* 1991; 248: 123.

[31] Cabero Ll, Escribano L, Cabero A, y cols. Acido palmítico e índice P/S en diabetes insulino-dependientes. *Clin Invest Ginecol Obstet* 1979; 6: 28.

[32] Korsud G, Balwin R. Effects of endocrinectomy and hormone replacement therapies upon enzyme activities in lactating rat mammary glands. *Biol Reprod* 1969; 1: 21.

[33] O'Sullivan JB. Gestational diabetes: factors influencing the rates of subsequent diabetes. In: Sutherland HV, Stowers JM, Eds. Carbohydrate metabolism in pregnancy and the newborn 1978. New York: Springer, 1979: 425.

Chapter 7

Long-term implications of gestational diabetes for the mother

David Hadden, Adele Kennedy, Ailish Nugent

David Hadden, MD FRCP, Consultant Physician and Honorary Professor of Endocrinology
Adele Kennedy, MD MRCP (UK), Specialist Registrar, Endocrinology and Diabetes
Ailish Nugent, MD MRCP (UK), Specialist Registrar, Endocrinology and Diabetes
Sir George E. Clark Metabolic Unit, Royal Victoria Hospital, Belfast BT12 6BA, United Kingdom.

Long-term implications of gestational diabetes for the mother

David Hadden*, Adele Kennedy, Ailish Nugent

Abstract.–Pregnancy in a normal woman is associated with physiological hyper-insulinaemia. These short-term changes in insulin synthesis and secretion are associated with pancreatic β cell hyperplasia and hypertrophy, which revert to normal after delivery. If the woman has some pre-existing disturbance of insulin action or β cell function, this will be exacerbated during the pregnancy and gestational hyperglycaemia or diabetes will occur. These women will be at greater risk of developing both Type 1 and Type 2 diabetes in the future. Increasing age, obesity and the degree of hyperglycaemia in pregnancy are risk factors for subsequent Type 2 diabetes. The presence of islet cell antibodies and glutamic acid decarboxylase (GAD) antibodies are predictive of Type 1 diabetes. Evidence that treatment of gestational diabetes during the pregnancy will lessen the risk of subsequent diabetes is inconclusive: there is some evidence that dietary, exercise and oral hypoglycaemic drug therapy after delivery will reduce the risk of diabetes.

Keywords: gestational diabetes, risk of type 2 diabetes, prevention of diabetes, is pregnancy diabetogenic?

*Address for correspondence: David Hadden MD FRCP, Consultant Physician and Honorary Professor of Endocrinology, The Queen's University of Belfast. Tel.: 028 90 894798, Fax: 028 90 310111

Introduction

Two main questions arise in discussion of gestational diabetes with a prospective mother. The old concept that pregnancy was diabetogenic is now largely discounted in epidemiological terms, although there are certainly short-term physiological adaptations which are in general advantageous to both mother and fetus, and interact with the control mechanisms for carbohydrate metabolism. More importantly there is broad agreement on the predictive value of blood glucose levels during the pregnancy not only for the growth and development of the fetus but also for the subsequent development of permanent diabetes mellitus in the mother. Gestational diabetes is an important indicator of subsequent diabetes and allows preventive measures to be considered, although the long-term nature of the pathophysiology makes studies of effectiveness difficult.

Is pregnancy diabetogenic?

Profound metabolic changes occur in normal pregnancy in the mother which facilitate optimal growth of the fetus. These include a progressive decrease in insulin sensitivity and an associated increase in insulin secretion [1]. Maternal fat deposition and diversion of glucose to the fetus are facilitated in the postprandial state, with increased maternal lipolysis during the fasting state. The changes in insulin action during pregnancy are largely as a consequence of hormone production by the fetoplacental unit, particularly human placental lactogen and progesterone [2], but may be influenced to a lesser extent by increased maternal caloric intake and reduced physical activity.

To maintain normal glucose tolerance in pregnancy, insulin secretion must increase. Hyperinsulinaemia occurs in the normal pregnancy and is a consequence of increased synthesis and secretion of insulin rather than reduced clearance [3]. These changes in insulin synthesis and secretion are accompanied by pancreatic β cell hyperplasia and hypertrophy [4]. Women with insufficient pancreatic β cell reserve are unable to compensate for the reduced insulin sensitivity of pregnancy and display consequent abnormalities in carbohydrate, lipid and protein metabolism with deleterious effects for both mother and fetus. The pregnancy-related changes in insulin sensitivity reverse rapidly following delivery of the placenta, with subsequent improvement or normalisation of glucose tolerance in women with gestational diabetes.

The earliest reported case of diabetes in pregnancy was described by Bennewitz in his thesis for the degree of Doctorate of Medicine in Berlin in 1824, and summarised in the Edinburgh Medical Journal in 1828 [5]. He described a young woman with onset of "unquenchable thirst" and production of large quantities of urine during her fifth pregnancy. He extracted 2 oz (56.7 g) sugar from 16 lbs (7264 g) of her urine. The baby, weighing 12 lbs (5448 g) died intrapartum, presumably due to delay in the second stage of labour. Post-partum, her strength improved daily and the sugar disappeared from her urine. Bennewitz believed that diabetes was a symptom of, or somehow due to the pregnancy.

Although the pregnant state has short-term diabetogenic effects, whether pregnancy is diabetogenic in the long-term has been a controversial issue. Early diabetes epidemiologists suspected a role for pregnancy in the subsequent

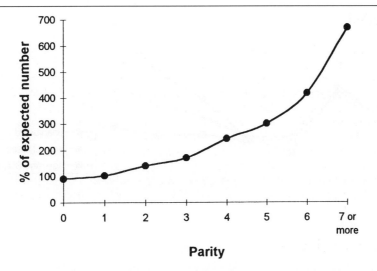

Figure 1. *Increase of incidence of diabetes with parity in women aged 45 or more. Expected number of women of each parity is calculated from a sample of the 1951 census of England and Wales* [8].

development of diabetes when they observed that the increased incidence of diabetes in female patients was accounted for by married women [6]. These observations were confirmed by others [7]. Pyke in London observed that parity and the difference in sex distribution in the general population together accounted for the then greater incidence of diabetes in women (*fig. 1*) [8]. He also reported an association between parity and obesity but found it insufficient to account for the relationship between parity and diabetes. Fitzgerald et al in Birmingham, UK confirmed an increased incidence of diabetes with increasing parity [9]. Compared to nulliparous women, they found those who had borne three children had a two-fold greater risk of diabetes, and those who had six or more children were six times more likely to have diabetes. They also reported an association between parity and obesity. More recently, a large prospective study examining the association between parity and subsequent development of diabetes has been reported in the USA [10]. The Nurses' Health Study cohort of 113,606 nurses aged 30-55 years without diabetes, coronary heart disease, stroke or cancer at enrolment were followed up for 12 years. There was an apparent association between parity and development of diabetes. However, following adjustment for age and body mass index, this association was completely abolished (*fig. 2*). This provides evidence that beyond its effect on bodyweight, parity has no independent effect on the risk of development of diabetes.

The change in pregnancy demography in many European countries in the past 50 years may also have had an effect on these relationships. In the large United Kingdom Prospective Diabetes Study of 5098 newly diagnosed Type 2 diabetic patients from 23 centres in the UK, only 2092 (two out of five) were female. Those of Asian or Afro-Caribbean ethnicity were younger and less overweight at diagnosis than the white Caucasians, but were more likely to have had three or more pregnancies by the time of diagnosis of their diabetes [11].

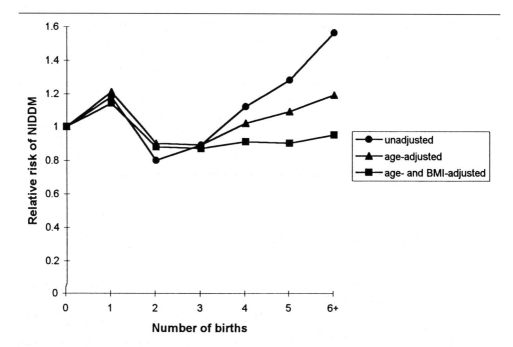

Figure 2. *Relative risk of NIDDM according to parity in a cohort of US women aged 30-55 years in 1976.*

The reference category is nulliparous women. The apparent positive association in unadjusted analyses is attenuated after adjustment for age and eliminated after adjustment for both age and BMI [10].

It has been suggested that gestational diabetes may merely represent detection of previously unrecognised impaired glucose tolerance. In a sample of 817 American women aged 20-44 years who were not pregnant and had no history of diabetes and who underwent a 75-g oral glucose tolerance test, a similar prevalence of both impaired glucose tolerance and of diabetes mellitus was demonstrated to those previously reported for gestational diabetes and gestational impaired glucose tolerance [12]. Although the conditions of testing for glucose tolerance were not uniform, this finding is compatible with the presence of impaired glucose tolerance or diabetes mellitus prior to pregnancy which is subsequently diagnosed during the routine testing during antenatal care, rather than an aetiological effect of pregnancy on these conditions. Routine screening for diabetes prior to pregnancy is not likely to become standard practice, but further population studies in this field would be useful.

It is well documented that gestational diabetes confers an increased risk of the subsequent development of diabetes. The identification of these patients provided the opportunity for targeting this high-risk group for primary prevention programmes. Although no long-term prospective studies of primary prevention of diabetes have been published, observational studies have demonstrated beneficial effects of physical exercise, weight control and low-fat diet on risk of diabetes, and there is evidence for the efficacy of primary prevention programmes in reducing the progression of impaired glucose tolerance to Type 2 diabetes [13]. The "Fasting Hyperglycaemia Study" in Oxford, in which patients with fasting plasma glucose levels in the range of 5.5 to 7.7 mmol/l (including patients with prior gestational diabetes) were randomised to treatment with either a sulphonylurea or placebo, reported that after one year those allocated to sulphonyl urea had significant reductions in fasting plasma glucose, HbA1c and improvement in β cell function [14]. Long-term studies of primary prevention in women with previous gestational diabetes using various therapeutic interventions are needed to determine how to manage these women who are at high risk for the future development of diabetes. Until such studies are available, these women should be advised to take regular physical exercise, maintain a healthy bodyweight and to consume a diet low in saturated fat.

Long-term implications of gestational diabetes for the mother

If pregnancy is considered as a short-term diabetogenic state manifested by increased insulin demands, caused by the increased secretion of hyperglycaemic hormones during pregnancy, gestational diabetes mellitus will occur when the pancreatic β cell function is insufficient to overcome the insulin resistance caused by the anti-insulin hormones, and by the increased fuel consumption required by the mother and the fetus [15]. Gestational diabetes mellitus has been defined as carbohydrate intolerance of varying severity, with onset or first recognition during pregnancy, irrespective of glycaemic status after pregnancy [16]. This definition although pragmatic and practical has the disadvantage of ignoring glycaemic status either before or after the pregnancy which makes precise classification impossible.

The prevalence of diabetes and of gestational diabetes varies considerably between, and within countries [17]. The incidence of gestational diabetes has been reported to be within 2-12% of all pregnancies. It varies according to age, obesity, race and family history of parental diabetes. There is unfortunately still international disagreement on the most appropriate diagnostic criteria. Some European studies have applied the World Health Organisation (WHO) criteria, but others have used the US National Diabetes Data Group (NDDG) criteria applied to a 75-g oral glucose tolerance test. Others have used the original Boston figures, with the use of a 100-g oral glucose load. It is obvious that higher the criteria for the diagnosis of gestational diabetes, the higher will be the risk of subsequent development of Type 2 diabetes. The large international HAPO (Hyperglycaemia and Adverse Pregnancy Outcome) study, using the 75-g oral glucose tolerance test, will finally establish a firm obstetrical baseline for plasma glucose in pregnancy.

Gestational diabetes has important short-term implications for the pregnant woman and her fetus and new-born infant. Longer-term consequences must also be considered, although in the majority of patients carbohydrate metabolism appears to return to normal immediately following delivery. The risk of developing overt diabetes or impaired glucose tolerance later in life is certainly increased. The incidence of subsequent Type 2 diabetes following gestational diabetes has been reported to be between 3 and 60% in various studies. *Table I* summarises studies published over the past 10 years. The figures vary

Table I. Follow-up studies of women with previous gestational diabetes.

Reference	City	Number	Diagnostic OGTT in pregnancy (g)	Follow-up	Diagnostic OGTT at follow-up	Abnormal glucose tolerance
Mestman	Los Angeles, USA	89	100	12-18 years	Interview	65% DM
Metzger et al	Chicago, USA	274	100	Up to 5 years	100 g (NDDG)	41% DM, 16% IGT
Dornhorst et al	London, UK	56	50	6-12 years	75 g (WHO)	39% DM, 25% IGT
O'Sullivan	Boston, USA	615	100	22-28 years	100 g (WHO)	36% DM
Damm et al	Copenhagen, Denmark	241	50	2-11 years	75 g (WHO)	3.7% Type 1 DM 13.7% Type 2 DM 17% IGT
Henry and Beischer	Melbourne, Australia	881	50	Up to 17 years	75 g (WHO)	12% DM, 16% IGT
Kjos et al	Los Angeles, USA	246	100	5-8 weeks	75 g (NDDG)	10% DM, 9% IGT
Coustan et al	Providence, USA	350	100	Up to 10 years	75 g (NDDG)	7% DM, 4% IGT
Persson et al	Stockholm, Sweden	145	50	3-4 years	75 g (WHO)	3.4% DM, 22% IGT
Hadden et al	Belfast, N Ireland	234	50	10 years	75 g (WHO)	0.5% DM, 2% IGT

DM, diabetes mellitus; IGT, impaired glucose tolerance; WHO, World Health Organisation; NDDG, National Diabetes Data Group (USA).

due to the fact that inhomogeneous populations have been studied, and diverging definitions and diagnostic tests for gestational diabetes have been used. There have also been different endpoint criteria for subsequent development of diabetes mellitus.

The longest follow-up study of women with gestational diabetes was undertaken in Boston, USA [32]. Six hundred and fifteen women with a history of gestational diabetes were followed, together with 328 controls (women with no gestational diabetes during pregnancy) for 22-28 years. The cumulative incidence of diabetes rose from 16% at 5 years after diagnosis to 40% at 15 years and reached 72% at 24 years, compared with 7% at 24 years in the controls (*fig. 3*). In the Boston study, a 100-g oral glucose load was used. To diagnose gestational diabetes, two or more venous glucose concentrations were required to equal or exceed a fasting value of 5.8 mmol/l, 1 hour value of 10.6 mmol/l, a 2-hour value of 9.2 mmol/l and a 3-hour value of 8.1 mmol/l.

One of the problems with comparisons between studies is the difference in the oral glucose load used in the individual studies. Comparison of the 75- and 100-g oral glucose loads showed that the 2-hour blood glucose value averaged 4 mg/dl

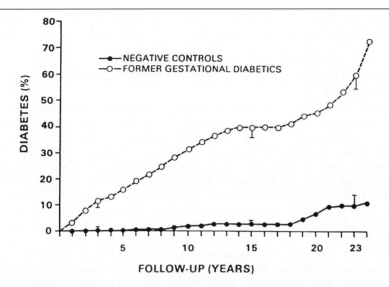

Figure 3. *Cumulative incidence of diabetes (per cent ± SE) in the Boston Gestational Diabetes Study* [32].

higher following the larger challenge [18]. An additional contributing factor to the differences in the incidence of gestational diabetes is the varying length of follow-up periods in the observational studies which ranged from 8 weeks to 28 years. In an Irish population, women with lesser degrees of glucose intolerance during pregnancy were not at an increased risk of developing glucose intolerance later in life [31]. Two hundred and thirty-four women were tested 10 years after delivery, who were traced from 625 mothers who had had a positive 50 g oral glucose tolerance test, and only six were abnormal and one diabetic. Mestman, however, in Los Angeles, USA, followed 360 Latino patients for up to 10 years [19] and showed that of those with an abnormal oral glucose tolerance test in pregnancy 13% became overtly diabetic, and a further 33% had abnormal tests 5 years after delivery. Latino women in the USA are an ethnic group known to be at an increased risk of developing diabetes. A study of 671 women with gestational diabetes who did not have diabetes after delivery showed within 7.5 years, using the 75-g oral glucose tolerance test, a 47% cumulative incidence rate of Type 2 diabetes [20].

In a cosmopolitan population in London, UK, both glucose tolerance and insulin secretion was studied in 56 women, 6-12 years following a pregnancy complicated by gestational diabetes, and in 23 matched controls [21]. The diagnosis of gestational diabetes had been made during the index pregnancy, using a 3-hour 50-g oral glucose tolerance test, whereas at recall a 75-g oral glucose load was used. The racial mix was Caucasian (35%), Asian, Afro-Caribbean, Middle-Eastern and Oriental, and the control group was of similar racial admixture. There was a high incidence of both overt Type 2 diabetes mellitus and impaired glucose tolerance using WHO criteria, approximately 60% of the study population had some abnormality of glucose tolerance within 12 years of the index pregnancy.

The incidence of Type 2 diabetes in the Pima Indian population is 19 times that in the general US population. Third trimester 2-hour post-load glucose concentration was evaluated in 233 women to predict diabetes 4-8 years after the index pregnancy. The proportion who developed diabetes increased with the glucose concentration, from 4.5% in those less than 5.6 mmol/l to 45.5% in those between 8.9 and 9.9 mmol/l [22].

Diabetes mellitus following gestational diabetes is typically thought to be Type 2 diabetes, but about 10% of the patients have circulating auto-antibodies to insulin or to islet cells [23]. This may well represent a latent form of Type 1 diabetes (LADA – Latent Autoimmune Diabetes with Autoantibodies). The risk of developing Type 1 diabetes following gestational diabetes has not been well established, but is probably greater in northern European countries where this type of diabetes is more prevalent. In a study in Copenhagen, Denmark, 2-11 years later in a group of former diet treated gestational diabetic women, 34% of 241 had developed abnormal glucose tolerance after 6 years, 3.4% were classified Type 1 diabetics, 13.4% as Type 2 diabetics and 17% as impaired glucose tolerance. The women who developed Type 1 diabetes had been younger and leaner during the index pregnancy, and tended to be diagnosed earlier following the pregnancy than those who developed Type 2 diabetes. A high prevalence was found of HLA DR3 and DR4 in addition to islet cell antibodies in the Type 1 group. In the Danish study the risk of Type 1 diabetes was approximately 20% [24].

Predictive factors for the development of overt diabetes in women with previous gestational diabetes

Gestational diabetes mellitus implies a significant risk to the mother for later development of overt diabetes. Not all women with hyperglycaemia during pregnancy do subsequently develop diabetes mellitus, so gestational diabetes may not always be a truly pre-diabetic state. However, gestational diabetes provides an opportunity for a primary screening programme for the prevention of diabetes and associated long-term complications. It is important to identify predictive factors to aid identification of those individuals who will develop diabetes in the future.

Several factors have been associated with the development of diabetes, which include obesity and age [25, 26, 27]; and the degree of hyperglycaemia during pregnancy [20, 24, 27]. In Copenhagen the fasting glucose value during pregnancy was an independent predictor for development of Type 2 diabetes [24] while in Californian Latino women the best prediction was from the area under the curve of the oral glucose tolerance test during pregnancy [20]. In Chicago, in women with previous gestational diabetes, the risk of developing diabetes rose from 23% when fasting glucose during pregnancy was less than 5.8 mmol/l to 86% when fasting glucose was greater than 7.2 mmol/l. Fasting glucose value could be used as a predictive factor when analysed as a continuous variable. The risk of subsequent diabetes was three times higher with a fasting glucose value of 5.6 mmol/l at diagnosis compared to a value of 4.7 mmol/l [27]. A poor insulin response to an oral glucose load during gestation has also been associated with an increased risk of diabetes in the long-term [24]. The presence of serum antibodies against glutamic acid decarboxylase (GAD65) in pregnancy was predictive of the development of Type 1 diabetes [23].

Despite the fundamental difficulties that arise when attempting to compare diabetes rates, there is a broad agreement on the predictive nature of the gestational glucose levels. Therefore, gestational hyperglycaemia, in addition to indicating a higher-risk pregnancy, will also indicate those individuals who are at increased risk of future diabetes. Gestational diabetes provides us with an opportunity for a primary screening programme for the amelioration or even prevention of diabetes and its associated long-term complications.

Prevention of diabetes following gestational diabetes

Some risk factors for subsequent diabetes are clearly unmodifiable. Ethnic group, age, family history of diabetes and even the degree of hyperglycaemia achieved in the pregnancy cannot be altered in a preventive strategy after the pregnancy. These programmes will have to concentrate on obesity and future weight gain, the composition of the diet and physical activity. There are a number of potential therapeutic substances, which may be useful, but clear evidence from randomised clinical trials is not available.

Obesity is the most important modifiable risk factor in women. Forty-one per cent of women enrolled in the UKPDS were above their ideal weight, compared to 21% of the men. Women with previous gestational diabetes are metabolically vulnerable and post-partum may still have impaired β cell function and insulin resistance to some degree. If they are still obese the risk of diabetes is much higher [27]. Weight loss will reduce insulin resistance, even if a relatively small reduction in actual weight is achieved – a 10-kg weight loss has been estimated to lessen the reduction in life expectancy of Type 2 diabetes by as much as 35% [28]. Obese women with previous gestational diabetes should receive advice on weight loss and non-obese women should strive to avoid weight gain. Dietary energy should contain less than 40% from fat, and a low fat/high complex carbohydrate formula will reduce insulin resistance. This dietary advice should be a logical extension of that given during the pregnancy.

Both short- and long-term physical activity will reduce insulin resistance by promoting muscle glucose uptake as well as by preventing adiposity. A prospective study of 80,000 non-diabetic middle-aged US women over 8 years showed that regular exercise reduced the risk of developing Type 2 diabetes by one-third [29]. The recommendation of the British Heart Foundation is to exercise for 20 minutes or more three times a week at 50% of the individuals maximum aerobic capacity which would represent brisk walking for most women over 45 years old.

The use of oral hypoglycaemic drugs to prevent progression of either β cell failure or of insulin resistance in patients at risk of Type 2 diabetes has so far been disappointing. Further randomised trials are in progress with metformin (which was the most effective therapy in the UKPDS protocol) and acarbose (which reduces disaccharide absorption), and also with new thiazolidinedione drugs which will increase insulin sensitivity.

References

[1] Buchanan TA, Metzger BE, Freinkel N, Bergman RN. Insulin sensitivity and beta-cell responsiveness to glucose during late pregnancy in lean and moderately obese women with normal glucose tolerance or mild gestational diabetes. *Am J Obstet Gynecol* 1990; 162: 1008-1014.

[2] Langhoff-Roos J, Wibell L, Gebre-Medhin M, Lindmark G. Placental hormones and maternal glucose tolerance: a study of fetal growth in normal pregnancy. *Br J Obstet Gynaecol* 1989; 96: 320-326.

[3] Bellman O, Hartman E. Influence of pregnancy on the kinetics of insulin. *Am J Obstet Gynecol* 1975; 122: 829-833.

[4] Van Assche FA, Aerts L, De Prins F. A morphological study of the endocrine pancreas in human pregnancy. *Br J Obstet Gynaecol* 1978; 85: 818-820.

[5] Bennewitz HG. Symptomatic diabetes mellitus (abstracted from Osann's 12ter Jahresbericht des Poliklinischen Institute zu Berlin, p23). *Edin Med J* 1828; 30: 217-218.

[6] Mosenthal HO, Boldoan C. Diabetes mellitus – problems of present day treatment. *Am J Med Sci* 1933; 186: 605-612.

[7] Monro HN, Eaton JC, Glen A. Survey of a Scottish diabetic clinic: a study of the aetiology of diabetes mellitus. *J Clin Endocrinol* 1949; 9: 48-78.

[8] Pyke DA. Parity and the incidence of diabetes. *Lancet* 1956; 1: 818-821.

[9] Fitzgerald MG, Malins JM, O'Sullivan DJ, Wall M. The effect of sex and parity on the incidence of diabetes mellitus. *Q J Med* 1961; 117: 57-70.

[10] Manson JE, Rimm EB, Colditz GA, Stampfer MJ, Willett WC, Arky RA et al. Parity and incidence of non-insulin-dependent diabetes mellitus. *Am J Med* 1992; 93: 13-18.

[11] UKPDS, UK Prospective Diabetes Study (12). Differences between Asian, Afro-Caribbean and white Caucasian Type 2 diabetic patients at diagnosis of diabetes. *Diabetic Med* 1994; 11: 670-677.

[12] Harris MI. Gestational diabetes may represent discovery of pre-existing glucose intolerance. *Diabetes Care* 1988; 11: 402-411.

[13] Eriksson KF, Lindgarde F. Prevention of Type 2 (non-insulin-dependent) diabetes mellitus by diet and physical exercise: the 6 year Malmo feasibility study. *Diabetologia* 1991; 34: 891-898.

[14] Karunakaran S, Hammersley MS, Morris RJ, Turner RC, Holman RR. The fasting hyperglycaemia study: III. Randomised controlled trial of sulfonylurea therapy in patients with increased but not diabetic fasting plasma glucose. *Metabolism* 1997; 46: 56-60.

[15] Freinkel N. Effects of the conceptus on maternal metabolism during pregnancy: on the nature and treatment of diabetes. *Excerpta Medica* 1965; 4: 679-691.

[16] The Third International Workshop Conference on Gestational Diabetes Mellitus. Summary and recommendations. 1991; 40(suppl 2): 197-201.

[17] Hadden DR. Geographic, ethnic and racial variations in the incidence of gestational diabetes mellitus. *Diabetes* 1995; 34:(suppl 2): 8-12.

[18] Castro A, Scott JP, Grettie DP, MacFarlane D, Bailey RE. Plasma insulin and glucose responses of healthy subjects and of varying glucose loads during 3-hour glucose tolerance tests. *Diabetes* 1970; 19: 842-851.

[19] Mestman JH. Follow-up studies in women with gestational diabetes mellitus. The experience at Los Angeles County/University of Southern California Medical Center. In: Weiss PAM, Coustan DR, Eds. Gestational diabetes. Vienna: Springer-Verlag, 1988: 191-198.

[20] Kjos SI, Peters RK, Xiang A, Henry OA, Monotoro M, Buchanan TA. Predicting future diabetes in Latino women with gestational diabetes: utility of early postpartum glucose tolerance testing. *Diabetes* 1995; 44: 586-591.

[21] Dornhorst A, Patterson CM, Nicholls JSD, Wadsworth J, Chiu DC, Elkeles RS et al. High prevalence of gestational diabetes in women from ethnic minority groups. *Diab Med* 1992; 9: 820-825.

[22] Pettittt DJ, Knowler WC, Baird R, Bennett PH. Gestational diabetes; infant and maternal complication of pregnancy in relation to third trimester glucose tolerance in the Pima Indians. *Diabetes Care* 1980; 3: 458-464.

[23] Damm P. Diabetes following gestational diabetes mellitus. In: Dornhorst A, Hadden DR., Eds. Diabetes and pregnancy: an international approach to diagnosis and management. Chichester: Wiley, 1996: 341-350.

[24] Damm P, Kuhl C, Bertelsen A, Molsted-Pederson L. Predictive factors for the development of diabetes in women with previous gestational diabetes mellitus. *Am J Obstet Gynecol* 1992; 167: 607-615.

[25] O'Sullivan JB. Body weight and subsequent diabetes. *JAMA* 1982; 248: 949-952.

[26] Catalano PM, Vargo KM, Bernstein IM, Amini SB. Incidence and risk factors associated with abnormal glucose tolerance in women with gestational diabetes mellitus. *Am J Obstet Gynecol* 1991; 165: 914-916.

[27] Metzger BE, Roston SM, Cho NH, Radvy R. Prepregnancy weight and antepartum insulin secretion predict glucose tolerance five years after gestational diabetes mellitus. *Diabetes Care* 1993; 16: 1598-1605.

[28] Goldstein DJ. Beneficial health effects of modest weight loss. *Int J Obesity* 1992; 16: 397-415.

[29] Manson JE, Rimm EB, Stampfer MJ et al. Physical activity and incidence of NIDDM women. *Lancet* 1991; 338: 774-778.

[30] O'Sullivan JB. The interaction between pregnancy, diabetes and long term maternal outcome. In: Reece EA, Coustan DR, Eds. Diabetes in pregnancy, principles and practice, 2nd edition. 1996: 389-397.

[31] Hadden DR. Screening for abnormalities of carbohydrate metabolism in pregnancy 1966-1997; the Belfast experience. *Diabetes Care* 1980; 3: 440-446.

[32] O'Sullivan JB. Diabetes mellitus after GDM. *Diabetes* 1991; 29:(suppl 2): 131-135.

Chapter 8

Infant of the diabetic mother

Bengt Persson, Ulf Hanson, Pauline Djerf

Bengt Persson, MD, PhD, Department of Women and Child Health, Karolinska Institute, Stockholm, Sweden.
Ulf Hanson, MD, PhD, Department of Obstetrics and Gynecology, University Hospital, Uppsala, Sweden.
Pauline Djerf, MD, Department of Obstetrics and Gynecology, Södersjukhuset, Stockholm, Sweden.

Infant of the diabetic mother*

Bengt Persson, Ulf Hanson, Pauline Djerf

Abstract.—Despite considerable improvement in the clinical management of the pregnant type 1 diabetic woman and her newborn, the incidence of foetal malformations is three times higher than in non-diabetics. Malformations are associated with much elevated HbA1c values (>8 SD above normal) during the embryonal period; recent data indicate that this threshold might be lower (i.e., >3-6 SD above normal). The incidence of macrosomia is 6-10 times higher than normal. Only a small fraction of the variation in birth weight can be explained by the level of glycaemic control during weeks 27-32. Other possible explanations for "unexplained" macrosomia could be that an exaggerated secretion of insulin, as well as other growth-promoting hormones (IGF1, 2), may be triggered by transient hyperglycaemia or by amino acids in early pregnancy. Other possibilities could be enhanced placental GLUT 1 activity and/or genetic factors. Neonatal hypoglycaemia includes a number of controversies related to analysis, definition, monitoring and short- and long-term consequences. Available data suggest that blood glucose values below 2.6 mmol/l beyond the first hours after birth may be harmful, provided appropriate techniques have been applied for specimen collection, processing and analysis of glucose. Long-term follow-up studies suggest that strict glycaemic control throughout gestation seems to protect the offspring from neurodevelopmental impairment. However, the risk for impaired glucose tolerance or diabetes and obesity increases later in life.

Keywords: type 1 diabetes mellitus, pregnancy, perinatal mortality, HbA1c, malformations, macrosomia, birth injury, neonatal hypoglycaemia, long-term prognosis.

---

*This article was accepted for publication in this volume in October 2001.

Introduction

The outlook for the offspring of the diabetic mother has never been brighter. The noticeable decline in perinatal mortality and morbidity rates during recent years can largely be attributed to improved blood glucose control before and during pregnancy. It is well recognised that foetal hyperinsulinism as a consequence of chronic maternal hyperglycaemia contributes to development of foetal macrosomia, delayed lung maturation and neonatal hypoglycaemia. It must be emphasised, however, that these and other morbidities have no single pathophysiological explanation. Several closely interrelated factors, such as acute pregnancy complications, degree of diabetic microangiopathy, gestational age and mode of delivery, will also influence foetal development and neonatal morbidity. As we have previously demonstrated, and as has been confirmed by others, prematurity per se significantly contributes to neonatal morbidity [1-3]. Despite the fact that major advances have been made in the clinical management of the pregnant diabetic and her newborn, we are still left with foetal and neonatal complications that may adversely influence the short- and/or long-term prognosis for the offspring. Several comprehensive reviews dealing with the newborn infant of the pre- or gestational diabetic mother have recently been published [4-6]. We have recently analysed the perinatal outcome of a large number of pregnancies complicated by type 1 diabetes in Sweden during the period 1991-96. This presentation focuses particularly on perinatal complications such as foetal malformations, foetal macrosomia, birth injury and asphyxia. We will also discuss some current controversies surrounding neonatal hypoglycaemia as well as some long-term follow-up results.

■ Foetal malformations

The incidence of foetal malformations in offspring of type 1 diabetic mothers is two to three times higher than in the non-diabetic population. The anomalies are not different from those seen in infants of non-diabetic mothers, with the exception of the caudal regression syndrome, which appears to be strongly associated with diabetes. Only a few studies have included a sufficient number of diabetic pregnancies and appropriate controls to allow for a meaningful analysis of the incidence of various types of malformations [7]. These studies suggest that the incidence of anomalies of the central nervous, cardiovascular, skeletal, genitourinary and gastrointestinal systems is greater in offspring of diabetic mothers than in those of non-diabetic mothers. Clinical and experimental data support the concept that poor metabolic control at the time of conception and organogenesis is an important teratogenic factor. Several studies have shown a significant association between elevated HbA1c in early pregnancy and the occurrence of foetal malformations and/or spontaneous abortion [8, 9]. It is important to underline that there is no relationship between elevated HbA1c and the severity of malformation. A significantly lower incidence (1.2%) of foetal malformations has been recorded in women who achieved strict glycaemic control during the pre-conceptional period compared with women whose blood glucose was well regulated only after the eighth week of gestation (10.9%) [10]. Similar findings have been reported by others and support the great importance of pre-pregnancy care.

During a prospective nationwide study conducted between 1982 and 85, defined to assess the relationship between HbA1c in early pregnancy (around week 9) and foetal malformation and/or spontaneous abortion, we found somewhat unexpectedly:

- that the incidence of major malformation was not significantly different from the corresponding national figure (2.0 vs. 1.75%, respectively), and
- that the incidence was significantly lower than that recorded (4.8%) in diabetic pregnancies during 1978-81 [8].

A similar decline in the malformation rate (from 7.2 to 3.1%) over approximately the same period was reported from Denmark [11]. In view of the significant association between an elevated HbA1c value and malformation, we speculated that the overall improvement in outcome could be attributed to the introduction of self-monitoring of blood glucose and multiple insulin injection therapy. Furthermore, a systematic education in pregnancy and diabetes for all adolescents with type 1 diabetes was initiated throughout the country in 1982.

A recent survey of all type 1 diabetic pregnancies ($n = 2463$) in Sweden during 1991-96 revealed a significant increase in the incidence of major malformations of 6.1% as compared to 1.9% in the non-diabetic population. Major malformations were defined as in our previous study 1982-85 [8]. There was no obvious explanation for this difference in the outcome during these two study periods. Unfortunately, the information concerning early pregnancy HbA1c values was not available during the 1991-96 study. It is thus possible that the higher incidence of malformations in the latter study is explained by less-rigid glycaemic control during the embryonal period. Of particular interest is a recent observation from an area in Southern Finland [12] which studied 709 infants of type 1 diabetic mothers and 735 controls born between 1988 and 97. The rate of major malformations was 4.2% versus 1.2% in the diabetic and control pregnancies, respectively. The authors confirmed that a much elevated HbA1c value (before week 14) was associated with foetal malformation, but also and more importantly, that only a moderate increase of HbA1c (i.e., 2-6 SD units above normal) was associated with an increased risk for malformation. The authors, in agreement with the recommendations of the American Diabetes Association, suggest that an upper optimal pre-pregnancy HbA1c level corresponds to the normal mean value + less than 3 SD units. Since the overall incidence of serious malformations is low, a large number of pregnancies are needed in order to detect changes in outcome over time. In order to further improve the management of diabetic pregnant women, there is an urgent need for nationwide, systematic registrations of the perinatal outcome including indices of the quality of glycaemic control.

Size at birth

The rate of foetal growth is determined by genetic, maternal, placental and foetal factors. Exactly how these factors interact is still not completely understood. In diabetic pregnancy, the foetal supply line may be altered in various ways. At one extreme, the supply line may be considerably reduced. This is a frequent complication in pregnant women with severe diabetic microangiopathy, in particular nephropathy. In this situation, uteroplacental blood flow is reduced with diminished placental transfer of substrates leading to intrauterine growth retardation. More frequently, the availability of substrates such as glucose and amino acids is significantly increased. Consequently, secretion and function of growth-promoting hormones like insulin, IGF 1 and 2 and their carrier proteins are exaggerated, leading to excessive transfer of nutrients and enhanced somatic growth. At birth these infants exhibit the classical features of a diabetic foetopathy with macrosomia and a plethoric and cushingoid appearance. Macrosomia is often defined as a birth weight >90th percentile for the gestational age and sex. However, we prefer the more stringent definition, i.e., a birth weight >2 SD. Meticulous control of maternal substrate levels by intensive insulin therapy may influence the foetal supply line and normalise the infant's size as well as appearance at birth. This favourable effect can to a large extent be attributed to a reduction of the adipose tissue mass, as indicated by significant correlation between the maternal glucose level during the last trimester of pregnancy and the skin-fold thickness and mean adipose cell diameter of the newborn (Whitelaw, 1977). No such relation exists between the maternal glucose level during the last 8-10 weeks of gestation and the birth weight (Persson, 1974). More recent studies have described a significant association between foetal macrosomia and either postprandial or fasting glucose values between weeks 29-32 and 27-32, respectively [13, 14]. It should be emphasised that this period of gestation coincides with the time of rapid foetal growth as determined by serial ultrasound measurements. Our study included a consecutive series of 113 pregnancies and was based on the analysis of daily self-monitored blood glucose determinations throughout pregnancy, each woman contributing with an average of 800 values. Both pre-pregnancy weight and fasting glucose values (between weeks 27 and 29) influenced the size of the infant. These two variables could, however, only explain around 12% of the variation in relative birth weight [14]. Despite intensive treatment with insulin, the rate of macrosomia was 26%, as in other reports.

A remarkable increase in the rate of macrosomia has occurred in Sweden from 20% (1983-85) to 33.5% (1991-96). Perinatal mortality dropped from 3.1 to 2.39% over the same time span. There is no apparent explanation for the higher rate of macrosomia. It must be emphasised, however, that a "tight" blood glucose control does not always result in normoglycaemia since the glycaemic goal must be raised sometimes in order to avoid severe hypoglycaemic episodes. Furthermore, foetal size decreases with increasing severity of diabetic angiopathy. A five-time reduction of diabetes nephropathy, and presumably incipient nephropathy, has been recorded in a recent Swedish study. Pre-eclampsia/pregnancy-induced hypertension, which is known to be closely associated with nephropathy, has also decreased from 20.6% (1983-85) to 13.8% (1991-96). Against this background, we have speculated that foetal growth restraining factors associated with severe diabetic microangiopathy may be less prevalent today than it was a few decades ago. Many centres have experienced the occasional and unexpected occurrence of foetal macrosomia despite very rigid control of maternal blood glucose. Both experimental and clinical data convincingly suggest that insulin per se plays a central role as regulator of foetal growth and development. The fact that newborns with nesidioblastosis or Beckwith's syndrome are macrosomic illustrates that foetal hyperinsulinaemia may enhance the transfer of glucose and other substrates from the mother to the foetus, despite the mother's being normoglycaemic. In diabetic pregnancy, it may well be that substrates other than glucose, such as branched-chain amino acids or insulin antibodies, stimulate foetal insulin production. Furthermore, we cannot exclude the possibility that an exaggerated β-cell function is already established at a very early stage of gestation [15], triggered by transient environmental changes in glucose and amino acids and/or genetic factors [16, 17]. Interestingly, elevated amniotic fluid insulin levels have already been recorded at 14-20 weeks gestation in women in whom gestational diabetes was later diagnosed (Carpenter et al, 1996). Another intriguing possibility to explain macrosomia, despite tight blood glucose control, is a significant increase of the placental glucose transporter GLUT 1 with a resultant close to 60% higher glucose uptake [18].

The typical diabetic foetopathy is characterised by increased amounts of total body protein, glycogen and fat; internal organs such as the liver, heart, adipose tissue, adrenals and pancreatic islet tissue are enlarged because of cellular hyperplasia and hypertrophy. This selective organomegaly contributes to a disharmonious body composition that may not be revealed by measurements of bodyweight and height. Abnormal growth of heart and adipose tissue can be assessed by non-invasive techniques. Increased thickness of the interventricular septum can be detected by echocardiography as early as 31-34 weeks gestation [19]. The prevalence of asymmetric septal hypertrophy is about 30%. This condition may present with or without symptoms. The amount of body fat that accumulates during the last 8-10 gestational weeks can be estimated using an anthropometric model that includes skin-fold measures [20]. In order to obtain a more balanced assessment of size at birth, it is suggested that measures of interventricular septal thickness (echocardiography) and adipose tissue mass (skin-fold calliper) should be performed. It is unlikely that leptin in cord blood can be used as an index of the amount of adipose tissue, as its concentration is also influenced by contribution from the placenta [21, 22].

Macrosomia and perinatal outcome

Macrosomia is associated with an increased risk of perinatal complications. A Swedish survey of type 1 diabetic pregnancies (1991-96) included 825 large (birth weight >2 SD), 1587 appropriate and 51 small for gestational age infants. The average gestational age of macrosomic foetuses was 38.0 as compared to 39.0 weeks, and as expected they were more often delivered by elective caesarean section (26.5% vs. 21.9%). Total perinatal mortality (2.9%) was 1.5 times and intrauterine death 2 times higher in the macrosomic infants as compared to the average-sized group of infants. Protracted labour, shoulder dystocia and birth trauma are well-known complications associated with vaginal delivery of the macrosomic infant. The incidence of plexus injury (5.5%) and clavicle fracture (8.4%) was almost 7 and 3 times higher than in the other group of infants. Contrary to other reports, there was no group difference in frequency of low Apgar scores (asphyxia). On the other hand, the incidence of symptomatic hypoglycaemia was significantly higher in the macrosomic group (10.7% vs. 5.7%). The association between foetal growth acceleration and neonatal hypoglycaemia illustrates the adverse consequences of foetal and subsequent neonatal hyperinsulinaemia.

Neonatal hypoglycaemia

The noticeable decline in circulating glucose concentrations after delivery, and particularly during the first hours after birth, is generally attributed to neonatal hyperinsulinaemia elicited by chronic maternal-foetal hyperglycaemia during pregnancy and/or labour and delivery. In newborns of diabetic mothers and controls, we recorded a nadir in plasma glucose concentration at 60 minutes after birth (1.2 vs. 2.8 mmol/l) and at 120 minutes, where values increased significantly (1.6 vs. 3.3 mmol/l) [23]. While profound hypo-glycaemia during the first hours after birth is frequently asymptomatic, clinical signs and symptoms often accompany similarly low glucose values at a later age. This different response to hypoglycaemia is not likely due to differences in the energy demands of the central nervous system (CNS), but is rather explained by the availability of alternate substrates such as lactate during the immediate neonatal period [24]. The possible functional role of glycogen stored in the CNS (astrocytes) is unknown. Newborn cats and dogs have three to four times higher concentrations of glycogen in the spinal cord and medulla of the brain as compared to adult animals. We speculated that this might also apply to humans and that infants of diabetic mothers have higher than normal glycogen levels in the CNS similar to that demonstrated in other organs. This could help explain a seemingly increased tolerance to hypoglycaemia and inappropriate counter-regulatory hormonal responses to hypoglycaemia in newborns of diabetic mothers.

The hormonal response (i.e., fail of insulin and rise of glucagon) to the physiological drop of blood glucose after birth, concomitant with a marked increase of TSH, favours metabolic adjustment by enhancing hepatic glucose production, lipolysis, fatty acid oxidation and ketogenesis. Reduced or normal glucose production rates during the first postnatal hours have been reported [25-27]. These variations can likely be attributed to differences in the quality of maternal glucose control during pregnancy [28]. Lipolysis, as reflected by a significant rise of plasma glycerol or as determined by the stable isotope technique, is not different from normal. When considering the interrelationship between the glucose disappearance rate and the lipid parameters determined at 2 hours after birth, our analysis indicated that lipolysis and the availability of plasma FFA decreased with an increasing degree of functional hyperinsulinism, as could be expected (Persson et al, 1976).

The subject of neonatal hypoglycaemia in general includes a number of controversial issues. Some of these controversies, such as the biochemical definition of hypoglycaemia, methods of monitoring blood glucose and the short- and long-term consequences, have recently been reviewed [29]. Since newborns of diabetic mothers are at increased risk of developing hypo-glycaemia and since the incidence of hypoglycaemia is considered an important outcome variable, it is appropriate to consider these questions in more detail.

■ Glucose analysis

In order to define the pre-analytical and analytical lower and upper normal levels of glucose, the following factors must be considered.

Pre-analytical factors

The accuracy and precision of the analytical method will depend on appropriate specimen collection and sample processing techniques.

■ *Sample source*

Capillary and arterial samples are approximately 10% higher than venous blood samples; plasma values are approximately 15% higher than venous blood values.

■ *Sample preservatives*

The rate of glycolysis within blood cells from newborn infants is much higher than in adults. In order to prevent falsely low glucose concentrations, samples should be collected into sodium fluoride (116 mg/ml) containing tubes and kept in ice water until centrifugation/or analysis. When using sodium iodoacetate as a preservative, significantly elevated blood glucose concentrations have been found with the Yellow Spring Instrument (YSI).

■ *Analytical factors*

Isopropyl alcohol (skin cleansing) should be avoided as it may interfere with the assay. Test strips and reflectance meters have caused much confusion; results are unreliable and cannot be used for diagnostic purposes. The HemoCue technique for whole blood seems to give more reproducible results, while values determined by wet chemistry are consistently lower.

■ Definition of neonatal hypoglycaemia

As was recently reviewed, different approaches to define neonatal hypoglycaemia have been applied [29].

■ *Level of blood glucose at which symptoms occur*

This definition may be questioned; symptoms are unspecific and some infants are asymptomatic (see above). A more useful definition is Whipples' triad: (1) low blood glucose, (2) symptoms, (3) symptoms disappear following the administration of glucose.

■ *Statistical definition*

Based on large numbers of glucose determinations in infants during the first postnatal days, hypoglycaemia could be defined as values outside −2 or −3 SD of the mean value for the age. Reference data published two or more decades ago are no longer applicable because of the improvement in care and management of newborns in recent years. According to more recently obtained results, a blood glucose level that is below 2.6 mmol/l is rarely observed in term or preterm infants during the first 24-48 hours after birth [29].

■ *Neurophysiological definition*

Abnormalities in brainstem auditory-evoked responses and somatosensory-evoked potentials were recorded in a small group of infants when blood glucose concentrations fell below 2.6 mmol/l; none of these infants had symptoms. The neurophysiological abnormalities disappeared or continued for many hours following restoration of normoglycaemia. We are not aware of any similar studies in offspring of diabetic mothers with asymptomatic hypoglycaemia (glucose <2.6 mmol/l) aged 24 hours or more. Cerebral blood flow is increased in premature infants with blood glucose <1.7 mmol/l and returns to normal following restoration of normoglycaemia [30]. This compensatory mechanism may explain the absence of symptoms in some infants with hypoglycaemia.

■ *Neurological outcome*

A large retrospective study of 661 preterm infants disclosed that infants whose blood glucose values were below 2.6 mmol/l five or more days during the neonatal period had a poor neurological outcome with increased incidence of developmental delay and cerebral palsy at the age of 18 months [31]. Subsequent follow-up studies at age 7.5-8 years have shown an association between neonatal hypoglycaemia and lower test scores for arithmetic and motor performance [32].

■ Clinical management

Prevention

In order to prevent the development of neonatal hypoglycaemia in infants of diabetic mothers, the following measures should be considered.

– Keep maternal blood glucose as close as possible to normal during pregnancy and, above all, maintain a glucose level around 4.5-5 mmol/l during delivery by adjusting injections of rapid-acting insulin or insulin infusion according to frequently measured blood glucose values.
– Reduce the infant's energy expenditure by preventing unnecessary heat loss immediately after birth and by keeping the infant in the thermoneutral zone. Consider administration of glucagon (200-300 µg/kg bodyweight) if blood glucose is low at a few hours after birth (i.e., <1.6-1.9 mmol/l), also in the absence of symptoms. Initiate early feeding (enteral or iv) aiming at full caloric intake at 3-4 days of age.

Detection

Monitor the blood (plasma) glucose, with first determination at 2-4 hours after birth, and thereafter every 3-4 hours before meals during the first 24-48 hours after birth. More frequent measurements may be indicated if there are additional risk factors such as poor metabolic control during pregnancy and delivery, prematurity, asphyxia, birth trauma, sepsis, macrosomia with typical appearance of diabetic foetopathy or feeding problems.

Diagnosis and treatment

If the infant exhibits symptoms such as jitteriness, convulsions, apneic spells, cyanosis, limpness, abnormal cry or bradycardia, and the blood glucose is below 2.6 mmol/l, intravenous glucose should be administered at an initial rate of

5 mg/kg and min. (equal to 3 ml of a 10% glucose solution/kg and min.). Continue with enteral feeds. If symptoms and/or low blood glucose values remain, the glucose infusion rate may be increased up to 10 mg/kg and min. If the glucose requirement is high, use more concentrated glucose solutions and administer into a central vein. If the infant has two or more blood glucose values below 2.2-2.6 mmol/l without symptoms, despite extra peroral intake, consider administration of glucagon and/or glucose infusion as above.

We fully agree with the expanded definition of hypoglycaemia proposed by Ansley-Green and Hawdon [29] as "the lowest concentration of glucose, which in combination with other metabolic fuels allows normal brain function". It is desirable that every nursery be equipped with a fast and accurate technique for bedside monitoring of blood glucose (e.g., Yellow Springs Instrument analyser), and that lactate (method available) and ketone bodies (3-hydroxy-butyrate) be simultaneously determined using micro-methods suitable for bedside analysis. Simple, reliable techniques for monitoring brain function are eagerly awaited.

Long-term prognosis

Infants of diabetic mothers are at increased risk of perinatal complications that may adversely influence the long-term prognosis. The marked reduction of perinatal mortality and morbidity rates in recent years implies that results of several studies published some decades ago are no longer representative of the present situation. There have been surprisingly few follow-up studies in recent years. In addition, methods used to assess morbidity vary, as well as the question of whether or not appropriate controls were included. Studies have mainly focused on two aspects: the future risk of developing diabetes and the neuropsychological development.

■ Future risk of developing diabetes

Children of parents with either type 1 or type 2 diabetes have an increased genetic susceptibility to developing impaired glucose tolerance (IGT) and/or diabetes. For unknown reasons, the incidence of type 1 diabetes is approximately five times higher in offspring of fathers (6.1%) as compared to mothers (1.3%) having type 1 diabetes [33]. Some ethnic groups, such as the Pima Indians, have a very high rate of type 2 diabetes that may already be diagnosed at an early age. Obesity, which is very prevalent in this population, represents an additional very significant risk factor for type 2 diabetes. The observation that a diabetic foetal environment per se accelerates the development of obesity and IGT/diabetes in the offspring is of considerable clinical importance [34]. Similar findings of a significantly increased incidence of IGT (19.3% vs. 2.4% in controls) was recently described in a racially mixed group of 10-16 year-old children of diabetic mothers [35]. This data should be interpreted with some caution as this study included the offspring of both type 1 and gestational diabetic women. Further studies are needed to clarify the interaction between foetal environmental and genetic factors, and to demonstrate whether improving the quality of glycaemic control during pregnancy can prevent the early onset of IGT/diabetes.

■ Neuropsychological development

A very high prevalence of neurological deficit and/or mental retardation has been reported in the past. However, subsequent studies have shown a much-improved outcome. Our follow-up of children of type 1 diabetic mothers at 5 years showed normal IQ scores without any relationship to maternal acetonuria during pregnancy, foetal size at birth or neonatal hypoglycaemia during the first hours after birth [36]. The importance of the level of glycaemic control in early pregnancy for the subsequent development of the offspring is indicated by an association between early foetal growth delay, as determined by ultrasonography between weeks 8 and 12, and delayed psychomotor development at 4 years of age [37]. More recent prospective studies of children of mothers with pre- or gestational diabetes demonstrated an essentially normal intellectual development when assessed at 2-5 years of age [38, 39].

References

[1] Hanson U, Persson B, Stangenberg M. Factors influencing neonatal morbidity in diabetic pregnancy. *Diabetes Res* 1986; 3: 71-76.

[2] Hanson U, Persson B. Outcome of pregnancies complicated by type 1 insulin-dependent diabetes in Sweden: acute pregnancy complications, neonatal mortality and morbidity. *Am J Perinatol* 1993; 10: 330-333.

[3] Hunter DJS, Burrows RF, Mohide PT, Whyte RK. Influence of maternal insulin-dependent diabetes mellitus on neonatal morbidity. *Can Mod Assoc J* 1993; 149: 47-52.

[4] Hod M, Diamant YZ. The offspring of a diabetic mother, short- and long-range implications. *Isr J Med Sci* 1992; 28: 81-86.

[5] Reece AE, Homko CJ. Infant of the diabetic mother. *Semin Perinatol* 1994; 18: 459-469.

[6] Persson B, Hanson U. Neonatal morbidities in gestational diabetes mellitus. *Diabetes Care* 1998; 21(suppl 2): 79-84.

[7] Mills J. Malformations in infants of diabetic mothers. *Teratology* 1982; 25: 385-394.

[8] Hanson U, Persson B, Thunell S. Relationship between haemoglobin A1c in early type 1 (insulin dependent) diabetic pregnancy and the occurrence of spontaneous abortion and foetal malformation in Sweden. *Diabetologia* 1990; 33: 100-104.

[9] Miodovnik M, Mimouni F, Tsang RC, Ammar E, Kaplan L, Siddiqi TA. Glycemic control and spontaneous abortion in insulin-dependent diabetic women. *Obstet Gynecol* 1986; 68: 366-369.

[10] Kitzmiller JL, Gavin LA, Gin GD, Javonovic-Peterson L, Main EK, Zigrang WD. Preconception care of diabetes glycemic control prevents congenital anomalies. *JAMA* 1991; 265: 731-736.

[11] Damm P, Mölsted-Pedersen L. Significant decrease in congenital malformation in newborn infants of an unselected population of diabetic women. *Am J Obstet Gynecol* 1989; 161: 1163-1167.

[12] Suhonen L, Hillesmaa V, Teramo K. Glycaemic control during early pregnancy and foetal malformations in women with type 1 diabetes mellitus. *Diabetologia* 2000; 33: 79-82.

[13] Coombs CA, Gunderson E, Kitzmiller JL, Gavin T, Main EK. Relationship of foetal macrosomia to maternal postprandial glucose control during pregnancy. *Diabetes Care* 1992; 15: 1251-1257.

[14] Persson B, Hanson U. Foetal size at birth in relation to quality of blood glucose control in pregnancies complicated by pregestational diabetes mellitus. *Br J Obstet Gynecol* 1996; 103: 427-433.

[15] Reiher H, Fuhrmann K, Noack W. et al. Age-dependent insulin secretion of the endocrine pancreas in vitro from fetuses of diabetic and non-diabetic patients. *Diabetes Care* 1983; 6: 446-451.

[16] Dunger DB, Ong KKL, Huxtable SJ, Sherriff A, Woods KA, Ahmed ML et al. Association of the INS VNTR with size at birth. *Lett Nat Genet* 1998; 19: 98-100.

[17] Gloria-Bottini F, Gerlini G, Lucarini N, Amante A, Lucarelli P, Borgiani P et al. Both maternal and foetal genetic factors contribute to macrosomia of diabetic pregnancy. *Hum Hered* 1994; 44: 24-30.

[18] Jansson T, Wennergren M, Powell TL. Placental glucose transport and GLUT 1 expression in insulin-dependent diabetes. *Am J Obstet Gynecol* 1999; 180: 163-168.

[19] Cooper MJ, Enderlein MA, Tarnoff H, Roge CL. Asymmetric septal hypertrophy in infants of diabetic mothers. Foetal echocardiography and the impact of maternal diabetic control. *AJDC* 1992; 146: 226-229.

[20] Catalano PM, Thomas AJ, Avallone DA, Amini SB. Anthropometric estimation of neonatal composition. *Am J Obstet Gynecol* 1995; 173: 1176-1181.

[21] Lepercq J, Cuazac M, Lablou N, Timisit J, Girard J, Auwerx J et al. Rapid publication. Overexpression of placental leption in diabetic pregnancy. *Diabetes* 1998; 47: 847-850.

[22] Persson B, Westgren M, Celsi G, Nord E, Örtqvist E. Leptin concentrations in cord blood in normal newborn infants and offspring of diabetic mothers. *Horm Metab Res* 1999; 31: 467-471.

[23] Persson B, Gentz J, Kellum M. Metabolic observations in infants of strictly controlled diabetic mothers. *Acta Paediat Scand* 1973; 62: 465-473.

[24] Vannucci R. Perinatal brain metabolism. In: Richard Polin, William Fox, Eds. Foetal and neonatal physiology, volume 2. Saunders, 1992: 1510-1519.

[25] Cowett RM, Susa JB, Giletti B, Oh W, Schwartz R. Glucose kinetics in infants of diabetic mothers. *Am J Obstet Gynecol* 1983; 146: 781-786.

[26] Kalhan SC, Savin SM, Adam PAJ. Attenuated glucose production rate in newborn infants of insulin-dependent diabetic mothers. *N Engl J Med* 1977; 296: 375-376.

[27] King KC, Tserng KY, Kalhan SC. Regulation of glucose production in newborn infants of diabetic mothers. *Pediatr Res* 1982; 16: 608-612.

[28] Baarsma R, Reijngoud DJ, Van Asselt WA, Van Doormaal JJ, Berger R, Okken A. Postnatal glucose kinetics in newborns of tightly controlled insulin-dependent diabetic mothers. *Ped Res* 1993; 34: 443-447.

[29] Ansley-Green A, Hawdon JM. Hypoglycaemia in the neonate: current controversies. *Acta Paediatr Jpn* 1997; 39(suppl 1): 12-16.

[30] Pryds O, Greisen G, Friis-Hansen B. Compensatory increase in CBF in preterm infants during hypoglycemia. *Acta Paediat Scand* 1988; 77: 632-637.

[31] Lucas A, Morley R, Cole TJ. Adverse neurodevelopmental outcome of moderate hypoglycaemia. *BMJ* 1988; 297: 1304-1308.

[32] Lucas A, Morley R. Letters Reply. Outcome of neonatal hypoglycaemia. *BMJ* 1999; 318: 194.

[33] Warram JH, Krolewski AS, Gottlieb MS, Kahn CR. Differences in risk of insulin-dependent diabetes in offspring of diabetic mothers and diabetic fathers. *N Engl J Med* 1984; 311: 149-152.

[34] Pettitt DJ, Nelson RG, Saad MF, Bennett PH, Knowler WC. Diabetes and obesity in the offspring of Pima Indian women with diabetes during pregnancy. *Diabetes Care* 1993; 16(suppl 1): 310-314.

[35] Silverman BL, Cho NH, Metzger BE, Loeb CA. Impaired glucose tolerance in adolescent offspring of diabetic mothers. *Diabetes Care* 1995; 18: 611-617.

[36] Persson B, Gentz J. Follow-up of children of insulin-dependent and gestational diabetic mothers. *Acta Paediat Scand* 1984; 73: 349-358.

[37] Petersen MB, Pedersen SA, Greisen G, Pedersen JF, Mölsted-Pedersen L. Early growth delay in diabetic pregnancy: relation to psychomotor development at age 4. *Br Med J* 1988; 296: 598-600.

[38] Rizzo TA, Ogata ES, Dooley S, Metzger BE, Cho NH. Perinatal complications and cognitive development in 2- to 5-year-old children of diabetic mothers. *Am J Obset Gynecol* 1994; 171: 706-713.

[39] Sells JC, Robinson NM, Brown Z, Knopp RH. Long-term developmental follow-up of infants of diabetic mothers. *J Pediatr* 1994; 125: 9-17.

Chapter 9

Lessons from experimental research: lasting consequences of fetal development in an abnormal intra-uterine milieu

Kathleen Holemans, Leona Aerts

Leona Aerts, PhD
Kathleen Holemans, PhD
Department of Obstetrics and Gynaecology, U.Z. Gasthuisberg, K.U.Leuven, Belgium.

Lessons from experimental research: lasting consequences of fetal development in an abnormal intra-uterine milieu

Kathleen Holemans, Leona Aerts

Abstract.–The mammalian fetus develops inside the uterus of its mother and is completely dependent on the nutrients supplied by the mother. Disturbances in the maternal metabolism that alter this nutrient supply therefore can induce structural and functional changes in the fetus, with lasting consequences for growth and metabolism of the offspring throughout life. This effect has been investigated in different experimental models by several research groups. The present chapter aims to compare the results of four rat models, in which the maternal metabolism was experimentally manipulated and the effect on the offspring was investigated: mild maternal diabetes during pregnancy, severe maternal diabetes, low protein diet and semistarvation of the mother. In each group altered fetal metabolism was associated with metabolic disturbances in the adult offspring, although the characteristics of the effects were divergent.

Mother	Mild diabetes	Severe diabetes	Low protein diet	Semistarvation
Fetus	hyperinsulinemia/		hypoinsulinemia	
	macrosomia/		microsomia	
Adult	disturbed glucose metabolism			
Pregnant	gestational diabetes			

These experimental data are compared to results from epidemiological studies on infants of mothers suffering from diabetes or malnutrition during pregnancy.

It can be concluded that fetal development in an abnormal intra-uterine milieu can induce alterations in the fetal metabolism, with lasting consequences for the glucose tolerance of the offspring in adult life. The most marked effect is the development of gestational diabetes, thereby transmitting the diabetogenic tendency to the next generation.

Keywords: diabetic pregnancy, gestational diabetes, intra-uterine milieu, fetal development, glucose tolerance, insulin resistance, experimental models.

Introduction

The mammalian fetus develops inside the uterus of its mother and, for its growth and development, is completely dependent on the nutrients supplied by the mother. Abnormalities in the maternal metabolism that alter the nutrient supply from mother to fetus can therefore interfere with normal fetal development. Diabetes of the mother during pregnancy for instance confronts the fetus with an abundance of glucose, while severe malnutrition (quantitative or qualitative) of the mother reduces the nutrient supply to the fetus. One of the obvious parameters for evaluation of fetal development is weight at birth. In the last decade evidence has been gathered of a significant correlation between birth weight and health in adult life, mainly at the level of glucose tolerance and cardiovascular diseases [1-5]. The intra-uterine milieu in which the fetus develops, therefore appears to program to a certain extend the condition of the individual throughout life. This transgeneration effect has also been called "fetal origin of adult disease".

The impact of the maternal metabolism on fetal development, and its lasting consequences for later health, have been studied in several experimental models where the maternal metabolism was modulated. The present chapter aims to review data, obtained by different research groups, where fetal development in an abnormal intra-uterine milieu results in metabolic disturbances in adulthood. Each study starts from pregnant rats in which circulating fuels have been experimentally manipulated: *mild maternal diabetes* during pregnancy, *severe maternal diabetes, mothers fed a low protein diet* and *semistarvation of the mother*. The effect of these differences in maternal metabolism on fetal development, especially in relation to glucose metabolism and growth, are described and compared to normal development. Long-term consequences of fetal development in an abnormal intra-uterine milieu, especially in relation to glucose homeostasis, are described in the adult offspring and even in subsequent generations. Alterations seen in fetal and adult offspring in the different experimental models are compared to normal development. Also comparison of the results between the different experimental models gives insight into the inducing factors and the mechanisms that cause these adaptation.

Fetal development

■ Normal development

The main substrate for fetal development is glucose (80%), which is completely derived from the maternal circulation, and the main growth hormone for the fetus is the insulin secreted by its own islets of Langerhans, responsible for 50% of fetal weight [6]. Toward the end of pregnancy the fetus is capable of regulating autonomically its own glucose homeostasis. Not fetal glycemia, but fetal insulinemia is significantly correlated with maternal glycemia [7]. The fetal endocrine pancreas is organized by then in mantle islets, with a central core of insulin containing β-cells surrounded by a mantle of non-β-cells. These β-cells already coexpress GLUT2, the typical glucose transporter of β-cells [8]. During the last days of gestation, an explosive expansion of the mass of endocrine pancreas occurs, as well as a quick maturation of the β-cells.

When challenged by glucose or another stimulus, they respond by secreting insulin, in vivo and in vitro [9]. At term fetal insulinemia is higher than at any other stage in life. In order to profit from this abundance of insulin, the fetal tissues must be equipped to capture the insulin (by insulin receptors), to internalize and degrade it (postreceptor mechanisms), and to initiate glucose entry (GLUT) and metabolism (glucokinase). Insulin receptors are present, and internalization occurs in fetal tissues from day 17 of gestation. Maturation gradually proceeds and at term fetal tissues show an abundance of insulin receptors, an adult capacity to bind insulin, and a progressive maturation of the postreceptor processes [10]. This allows the fetus to profit maximally from the circulating nutrients for its growth and development, and especially for the spectacular increase in bodyweight in late gestation. Besides glucose, amino acids play an important role in fetal development. At one hand, amino acids are potent stimulators of the fetal endocrine pancreas, at the level of islet development as well as that of β-cell secretion [11, 12]. On the other hand, the high circulating insulin levels, originating from these fetal islets, promote the consumption of amino acids as building blocks and fuels [13]. Also the nonprotein amino acids, exerting their own metabolic function, play an important role in fetal development. Taurine, a neurotransmitter necessary for the proliferation and differentiation of the fetal brain cells, is an essential amino acid in fetal life. It is accumulated in the tissues of the pregnant mother, and fetal concentrations (very high in brain, liver and placenta) are depending on the placental transport [14, 15]. Taurine is abundant in the non-β-islet cells and might be involved in the paracrine/autocrine regulation of islet cells [16]. In vitro, taurine stimulates insulin secretion by fetal rat islets [17]. Circulating fetal insulin also can modulate organ development during late gestation. The fetal hypothalamus appears to be particularly sensitive to insulin. Increased insulin concentrations can permanently damage the structure and function of the ventro-medial nucleus, compromising thereby glucose metabolism throughout life [18].

■ Mild maternal diabetes

When the mother has mild diabetes (glycemia increased by ±20%) during pregnancy, induced by destroying part of the β-cells [9, 19] or by continuous glucose infusion [20], increased amounts of glucose reach the fetus by facilitated transport through the placenta. In order to deal with this abundant glucose supply, adaptations occur in fetal insulin production and insulin action. The development of the fetal islets of Langerhans is enhanced, resulting in hypertrophy of the endocrine pancreas and hyperplasia of the β-cells. Not only the number of fetal β-cells is increased, but also the biosynthetic activity of the individual insulin-producing cell is enhanced [19]. The insulin response to glucose stimulation, both in vivo and in vitro, is clearly increased in the fetuses of mildly diabetic mothers as compared to controls [9]. In cultured neonatal islets such an increased sensitivity appears to be associated with an increased presence of Glut2 on the β-cell membranes [21]. All these adaptations of the fetal endocrine pancreas to maternal diabetes result in fetal hyperinsulinemia. High levels of insulin are circulating in the fetus of the mildly diabetic mother in the last third of pregnancy, when maturation of the insulin receptors and postreceptor mechanisms occurs. In rabbit fetal tissues, it has been shown that such hyperinsulinemia in utero increases the number of insulin receptors [22] and in neonatal rats maturation of GLUT4 and expression of glucokinase is enhanced by a high-carbohydrate diet [8, 23]. In the MD fetuses, the combination of an excess of maternally derived glucose, fetal hyperinsulinemia, and an increased number of insulin receptors in the fetal tissues is in favor of accelerated glucose uptake. However, not only glucose utilization by the fetal tissues has altered, also amino acid turnover is involved. Even a short infusion of high insulin concentration at normal glucose level promotes the entry of glucose into fetal tissues, and also the uptake of amino acids and the protein synthesis [24]. In our experimental model, circulating amino acid levels are similar in control and mildly diabetic mothers. In the fetuses, however, amino acid levels are significantly lower in the MD fetuses than in controls, and this is a global effect involving almost all amino acids, essential and nonessential [25]. Since the supply of amino acids by the mother appears to be normal, the low levels in the fetus are in agreement with an increased AA uptake by the fetoplacental unit as a result of fetal hyperinsulinemia. Remarkably the concentrations for the nonprotein amino acid taurine (important for fetal brain development) are very low in MD mothers and fetuses. Fetal or neonatal hyperinsulinemia is known to have a deleterious effect on hypothalamic development [18]. Administration of insulin in the circulation, or directly into the hypothalamus, in the perinatal period results in hypoplasia of the ventro-medial nucleus and permanent disturbance of glucose homeostasis. These effects are described also in the hyperinsulinemic fetuses of mildly diabetic mothers. We can summarize that, in mild maternal diabetes, hyperglycemia stimulates the fetal endocrine pancreas to islet hypertrophy and β-cell hyperactivity. The consequential hyperinsulinemia and accelerated anabolism, involving the increased uptake of glucose and amino acids, result in fetal macrosomia. Alterations in the hypothalamic development, and in the presence of nonprotein neurotransmitters, might compromise the regulation of insulin secretion.

■ Severe maternal diabetes

When maternal rats are made severely diabetic (by destroying the majority of their β-cells), the fetuses are confronted with very high glucose concentrations. The severe fetal hyperglycemia induces islet hypertrophy and β-cell hyperactivity, and might result in early hyperinsulinemia. This adaptation however appears to be limited, β-cells are overstimulated and the secretion of insulin is faster than its biosynthesis. β-Cells become depleted of insulin and often appear dysorganized and almost depleted of insulin granules [19]. These degranulated cells are incapable of insulin secretion in vivo and in vitro [9] and β-cell exhaustion results in fetal hypoinsulinemia. The development of the insulin receptor and post-receptor system is thereby altered, receptors in fetal lung and liver are low [26], and glucose uptake [27] and protein synthesis [28] are decreased. Circulating AA levels in these SD fetuses are significantly lower than in the controls; in fact the fetal levels parallel the low maternal levels and the feto-maternal ratio is normal [25]. Taurine levels, however, are exceptionally low in mothers and fetuses. Despite the abundance of glucose, fetal anabolism is low, resulting in microsomia [9, 19]. In summary, in the fetuses of severely diabetic mothers, the extremely high glucose levels induce islet hypertrophy, overstimulation and disorganization of fetal β-cells, resulting in low circulating insulin levels and impaired development of the insulin-receptor system; fetal anabolism is stunted leading to microsomia.

■ Mothers on a low-protein diet

When pregnant rats are fed with an isocaloric low-protein diet throughout pregnancy (8% vs. 20% protein), maternal plasma glucose and insulin levels remain normal throughout pregnancy, but amino acid concentrations are altered. Despite fetal normoglycemia, the development of the fetal endocrine pancreas is impaired due to the combination of a decreased proliferative capacity and an increased apoptotic rate of the islet cells. At term, mean islet size is therefore significantly reduced, with a relatively smaller proportion of β-cells, resulting in a reduced total islet mass and insulin content and a deficient insulin response, at least in vitro. Vascularization of the islets is decreased, due to a lower number of blood vessels [29–32]. Plasma levels of several amino acids are low in these LP mothers and their fetuses, taurine being the most affected. Addition of taurine to the drinking water restores taurine levels in mothers and fetuses. The insulin release from the fetal islets after stimulation in vitro with taurine and other secretagogues is thereby restored [33]. The data confirm that amino acids are potent stimulators of pancreatic development and β-cell function. Although these mothers receive a normocaloric diet and are normoglycemic throughout pregnancy, the development and function of the endocrine pancreas of their fetuses is disturbed, and birth weight is significantly reduced [32].

■ Semistarvation of the mother

When maternal food intake is restricted to 50% of the normal consumption, from day 11 [34] or day 15 [35] of pregnancy, nonfasting plasma glucose and insulin concentrations are, respectively, 25 and 75% lower than in pregnant rats fed ad libitum. At term, the fetuses of these food-restricted rats are hypoglycemic and hypoinsulinemic and remain microsomic (80% of control weight). In the growth-retarded newborns, the number of pancreatic islets is reduced, and β-cell mass is significantly decreased, as well as pancreatic insulin content. Proliferative capacity of the β-cells, however, is not altered [36]. Severe food restriction of the mother leads to severe retardation in fetal growth and development, including structural and functional deficiency of the fetal islets of Langerhans.

■ Comparison between the experimental models

In the four experimental models described here, the alterations in maternal metabolism have altered the fuel supply from mother to fetus, inducing functional and structural adaptations during fetal development. The fetuses of mildly diabetic mothers have to deal with an increased glucose supply, inducing fetal hyperinsulinemia, resulting in an accelerated anabolism and macrosomia. The three other models produce newborns with intra-uterine growth retardation. In the fetuses of severely diabetic mothers, this microsomia, despite abundant glucose supply, is due to low insulin levels as a result of exhaustion of β-cell function. In the fetuses of malnourished mothers, the fuel supply itself is deficient, in a qualitative or a quantitative way, and prevents an adequate development of the fetal endocrine pancreas, resulting in hypo-insulinemia and low fetal anabolism.

Lasting consequences in the adult offspring

■ Normal development

After birth, neonatal feeding switches from maternally derived fuels rich in carbohydrates to maternal milk very poor in carbohydrates. Regarding the development of the endocrine pancreas, lactation appears to represent a steady-state period, since the mass of islet tissue and the activity of the β-cells hardly increase [19]. However, it has been shown recently that, on the contrary, a complete reorganization of the islets of Langerhans takes place postnatally. A wave of apoptosis occurs, counterbalanced by islet cell replication and neogenesis. The effect is situated in the β-cells; it occurs during normal development of the endocrine pancreas and results in a renewal (at least partly) of the β-cell population [37]. After weaning, the mass of endocrine pancreas relative to pancreas and bodyweight, decreases sharply; at adult age the volume density of islet tissue in the pancreas is limited to less than 1% versus some 5% in the perinatal period [19].

■ Mild maternal diabetes

No data are available yet on this postnatal reorganization in the hypertrophic islets of Langerhans of newborns from diabetic mothers. After withdrawal of the hyperglycemic maternal stimulus at birth, the lactation period appears to represent a poor stimulus for the further development of the endocrine pancreas, which ends up hypoplastic by the time of weaning [19]. However at adulthood, the youngsters of mildly diabetic mothers display a normal mass of endocrine pancreas, with a normal contribution of the different islet-cell types [38]. Glycemia and insulinemia are normal, at least in basal conditions. On glucose stimulation however, in vivo and in vitro, insulin response is deficient. In this and other experiments with perinatal hyperinsulinemia [18, 39-41], glucose tolerance in the adult animal is impaired [19]. This impairment in the adult youngsters can be induced by increasing endogenous or exogenous insulin levels in the fetal or neonatal plasma, or by administrating insulin directly into the perinatal hypothalamus. This fetal or neonatal hyperinsulinism is related with persistent hypoplasia of the hypothalamic ventro-medial nucleus, involved in the regulation of food intake and insulin secretion [18]. While basal plasma glucose levels are normal, amino acid concentrations are remarkably low in these offspring of mildly diabetic mothers at adult age, as they were during fetal life [25]. Again this effect is seen for each group of amino acids, and for almost each individual AA. The low levels of circulating AA as such, might explain at least partly the deficient insulin response on glucose stimulation in these animals, since preincubation of islets from MD youngsters with a mixture of amino acids restores normal insulin response [19]. The extremely low levels for taurine, mainly dependent on dietary intake [25] in these animals with normal food consumption, suggest an alteration in the turnover and/or accumulation of taurine in the tissues of these offspring. It can be summarized that adult offspring of mildly diabetic mothers, although normoglycemic in basal conditions, display an impaired glucose tolerance. The primary inducing factor probably is the fetal hyperinsulinemia, enhancing fuel uptake and metabolism in various tissues, and provoking permanent damage to the central nervous system involved in lifelong modulation of metabolism.

■ Severe maternal diabetes

Postnatal development of the microsomic pups born to severely diabetic mothers is retarded, and the animals remain small up to adulthood [19]. Data are not available on the postnatal reorganization of the endocrine pancreas, which remains small during the lactation period. At adult age, however, the endocrine pancreatic mass in these animals exceeds control values, and this excess of islet mass is due to a high number of very small islets of Langerhans [38], suggesting an increased contribution of β-cell neogenesis, rather than cell replication. Plasma amino acid concentrations are normal in the adult youngsters of severely diabetic mothers, including the levels for the neurotransmitters taurine, GABA and carnosine [25]. Nonfasting glucose and insulin levels again are normal in the adult youngsters, as well as the insulin sensitivity of the tissues in basal condition. In vivo and in vitro, stimulation of β-cells exerts an increased secretion of insulin [19]. Furthermore, the ability of insulin to stimulate glucose utilization, especially by the skeletal muscles, and to inhibit glucose production is decreased in these offspring [42, 43]. This insulin resistance can partly, but not completely, be restored by normalizing maternal glycemia with islet transplantation in the course, or even before, pregnancy [43]. Factors other than maternal hyperglycemia, present in the mother as a result of actual or former severe diabetes, must therefore be responsible for the induction of insulin resistance in this offspring. In this offspring of severely diabetic mothers, basal glucose homeostasis is normal, but challenging glucose tolerance is associated with hyperinsulinemia and insulin resistance in liver and peripheral tissues. Fluctuations in fetal hyperinsulinemia might have affected later insulin secretion via the hypothalamic pathway, but insulin resistance must be induced by factors other than maternal hyperglycemia per se.

■ Mothers on a low-protein diet

The microsomic newborns of mothers fed a low-protein diet during pregnancy and/or lactation continue to grow slowly during the lactation period, and at weaning they are significantly smaller than normal, the effect being most marked in pups also lactated by LP mothers [33, 44]. The size of most organs is reduced in proportion to the bodyweight, however some organs (pancreas and liver) are more affected, while others (brain and lung) are relatively protected. During the postnatal reorganization of the islet mass, an increased incidence of apoptosis is seen, combined with a reduced β-cell proliferation rate due to an altered length of the cell cycle. This results in a reduced total islet and β-cell mass, as well as insulin content [33]. When these pups are weaned on a low-protein diet, their bodyweight remains below normal, with a deficient mass of endocrine pancreas and a low pancreatic insulin content [30, 31]. Fasting plasma insulin levels are low, in the presence of normal glucose levels. During glucose stimulation, insulin response is deficient, due to metabolic abnormalities at the level of the islets [45], and glucose tolerance is clearly impaired. In basal condition, these youngsters display a specific marked decrease in pancreatic and islet blood flow. During a glucose challenge, however, the increase in islet blood flow is higher than normal in the LP youngsters, thereby reaching control values [46]. If fed a normal diet from birth until adulthood, recuperation is seen with regard to bodyweight, but the insulin secretory pattern is only partially restored and glucose metabolism remains impaired, especially in the female offspring [30, 31]. Organs size grossly keeps in proportion to the body mass, with persistent protection of the brain [44], while vascularization of the cerebral cortex remains deficient [47]. Specific protein deficiency of the mother during pregnancy, despite normoglycemia, induces not only neonatal but also permanent structural and functional deficiency of the endocrine pancreas in the offspring.

■ Semistarvation of the mother

In pups from mothers semistarvated during pregnancy and lactation, β-cell mass remains unchanged from birth to weaning, whereas it increases three-fold in control animals. The estimated β-cell number, already below normal at birth, reaches only 30% of the control value at weaning. The proliferation capacity of the β-cells however remains normal, suggesting an alteration at the level of cell differentiation and/or apoptosis [35]. Bodyweight remains significantly lower than normal [34, 35]. After weaning on a normal laboratory diet, the difference with control weights decreases, but is still significant at adulthood [34]. At 3 months of age, animals malnourished during their fetal and early postnatal life show a normal glycemic response to an oral glucose load, despite a significantly decreased insulin response [48]. Total β-cell mass and number are decreased by some 20%, despite a pronounced increase in cell proliferation rate, the difference being mainly situated in the head of the pancreas [35]. Peripheral glucose utilization remains normal in basal state and during hyperinsulinemia, but insulin responsiveness by the liver is decreased, accounting for the insulin resistance seen in these animals [34]. Blood pressure is normal, but subtle changes in vascular function are seen [48]. The situation gets worse with age; no further increase in bodyweight is seen after the age of 4 months, and at 8 months pancreatic insulin content is decreased by 40% [48]. Nonfasting plasma insulin levels are markedly decreased in these youngsters, resulting in mild hyperglycemia. At 12 months of age, fasting glycemia is increased and glucose tolerance is dramatically impaired with insulinopenia in basal and stimulated conditions [50]. Similar effects are seen in offspring of mothers semistarved during pregnancy only, not during lactation. Bodyweight in these offspring catches up very quickly and these animals become even heavier than controls [34]. Thus, global food restriction of the mother during pregnancy induces permanent metabolic alterations in the offspring, including decreased basal and stimulated insulin release and mild hyperglycemia. Insulin resistance is mild in these animals, and is confined to the liver [34].

■ Comparison between the experimental models

Especially from the experiments of Plagemann et al [18], it is clear that perinatal hyperinsulinemia, as in the macrosomic fetuses of mildly diabetic mothers, is the inducing factor for at least part of the metabolic disturbances in the adult offspring. The induced alterations in the development of the hypothalamus result in permanent hypoplasia of the ventro-medial nucleus, associated with impairment of stimulated insulin response. Besides its effect on the CNS, fetal hyperinsulinemia also initiates alterations in amino acid metabolism, that are specific for the youngsters of MD mothers, and that persist into adulthood. Also the resulting low plasma levels of almost all amino acids, including taurine, contribute to the deficient insulin response in these animals.

Comparing the offspring of the three animal models with growth-retarded fetuses, it is clear that microsomia at birth is associated with metabolic alterations in later life, but that the characteristics of these alterations are not similar between the groups. Whereas starvation during the neonatal period has no effect on the glucose uptake by the peripheral tissues, severe maternal diabetes significantly reduces glucose uptake by the skeletal muscles. Whole-body insulin resistance thereby is more pronounced in offspring of diabetic, than of semistarved mothers, where only a mild hepatic insulin resistance is seen. Perinatal growth retardation per se, comparable between the two groups, can therefore not be the cause of later peripheral insulin resistance. Also fetal hypo-insulinemia at term, the period of development of the insulin-receptor system, is not the factor inducing insulin resistance in the peripheral tissues. Insulin levels indeed are equally low in the fetuses of semistarved and in those of severely diabetic mothers, although the origin of these low levels is divergent. The insulin resistance in the peripheral tissues of the offspring of severely diabetic mothers must be induced by a factor, other than hyperglycemia, intrinsic to the diabetic state of the mother; the hyperresponsiveness of the β-cells in this offspring might result from this increased insulin need. The primary defect in the glucose regulation of offspring from malnourished mothers appears to be at the level of size and function of the endocrine pancreas; the mild insulin resistance in the liver may result from hypo-insulinemia itself.

Besides metabolic alterations, offspring of rats on a low-protein diet also have an increased blood pressure [50]. In both offspring of diabetic and of semistarved rats blood pressure is normal. Subtle changes in vascular function, however, have been demonstrated in adult offspring of semistarved rats [49], whereas vascular endothelial dysfunction is more pronounced in offspring of diabetic rats [52].

Transmission of the diabetogenic effect to the next generation

From the previous data it is clear that development of the fetus in an abnormal intra-uterine milieu can induce functional and structural adaptations, resulting in lasting consequences for the metabolism of the offspring throughout life. These alterations might not be obvious in basal conditions, but become apparent in situations stressing glucose metabolism. Pregnancy is a condition that puts great demands on maternal metabolism, and more specifically on insulin secretion and action. Deficient adaptation to the situation of pregnancy might result in gestational diabetes.

■ Normal pregnancy

During normal pregnancy plasma insulin concentrations increase very sharply, and plasma glucose decreases. This hyperinsulinemia of pregnancy is associated with adaptations at the level of the islets of Langerhans: there is a doubling of the total amount of endocrine pancreas, with a parallel doubling of the β-cells. On top of the increase in β-cell number, an increased activity in these β-cells is seen in basal condition [38, 53], and an increased sensitivity and responsiveness to stimuli. Normal pregnancy is also associated with insulin resistance. From the results of euglycemic hyperinsulinemic clamps, it can be seen that the effect of insulin on glucose metabolism decreases during pregnancy. This global insulin resistance is situated as well at the level of peripheral glucose consumption, as at the level of hepatic glucose production [54].

■ Mild maternal diabetes

In the adult youngsters of mildly diabetic mothers, the adaptation of the endocrine pancreas to pregnancy is comparable to that of the controls [38, 53], and circulating insulin levels also increase during pregnancy, however not to the same extent as in the controls. Glucose levels thereby do decrease, but again not to the same extent as in the controls, resulting in a mild but significant hyperglycemia, due to an impaired adaptation to the situation of pregnancy: this is gestational diabetes. This means that the fetuses of these youngsters also develop in the abnormal intra-uterine milieu of a mildly diabetic mother, and indeed they do display the typical features of MD fetuses: macrosomia, islet hyperplasia and β-cell degranulation. When they become adult, they have an impaired glucose tolerance with the same characteristics as offspring of MD mothers [19, 39, 41]. The diabetogenic effect is thereby transmitted to the next generation. This transgeneration effect into the third generation, fetuses and adults, is only transmitted via the maternal line: female offspring of diabetic mothers develop gestational diabetes and induce the effect in their fetuses, and thereby in the next generation. Male offspring have impaired glucose tolerance, but do not transmit the effect to their offspring [19]. This observation stresses again the impact of the maternal environment and excludes a genetic interference.

■ Severe maternal diabetes

In the nonpregnant youngsters of the SD mothers, the total amount of islet mass is excessive, while islet composition is normal. The increase in total islet mass during pregnancy is not significant, but since this was already high, it reaches the level of the normal situation during pregnancy [38]. In the offspring of the SD mothers, insulin resistance is already present without pregnancy and does not increase further during gestation [55]. Nevertheless, as in the MD youngsters, circulating insulin does not increase to the same level as in normal pregnancy, and also the pregnant youngsters of severely diabetic mothers develop gestational diabetes. Their fetuses thereby also develop in the intra-uterine milieu of a mildly diabetic mother, and their offspring display the typical features of offspring from mildly diabetic mothers, as fetuses and as adult youngsters [19]. Also here, a diabetogenic tendency is transmitted to the next generation, as a result of fetal development in a diabetic mother.

■ Mothers on a low-protein diet

When adult female offspring of mothers fed a low-protein diet become pregnant, they display fasting hyperglycemia and impaired glucose tolerance. Insulin response on glucose challenge is deficient, whether the low-protein diet was continued during lactation and up to adult age, or just restricted to the gestational period. The fetuses, developing in these mildly hyperglycemic mothers, display a significantly higher pancreatic insulin content [30], possibly related to islet hyperplasia. Also in this experimental model, the low-protein diet of the first generation mother, especially during pregnancy, results in a diabetogenic condition in her offspring, with consequences for the subsequent generation.

■ Semistarvation of the mother

When adult youngsters of semistarved mothers become pregnant at the age of 4 months, they are able to double their islet mass and to increase significantly the insulin content of their islets as it occurs in normal pregnancies. At older age however (8 months), pancreatic insulin content, already half of the normal value before pregnancy, hardly increases during pregnancy and islet mass remains similar to nonpregnant values throughout pregnancy. This is associated with a deficient islet number rather than islet size [48]. Early malnutrition therefore appears to have dramatic consequences on the capacity of the endocrine pancreas to meet the increased insulin demands of pregnancy, certainly at older age.

■ Comparison between the experimental models

Pregnant offspring of mildly and severely diabetic mothers have the appropriate equipment for insulin production and secretion as compared to normal pregnancy. Also, insulin resistance is comparable to that of normal pregnancy. These features, however, are already present before pregnancy, and further pregnancy-induced adaptations are absent. Consequently, a gestational diabetes develops in these pregnant offspring.

Malnutrition of the mother during pregnancy, on the contrary, appears to have a deleterious effect on the development of the endocrine pancreas of the youngsters throughout life. Deficient islet mass and β-cell activity, already significant without pregnancy, deteriorates during gestation. Gestational diabetes in these animals appear to result primarily from insulin deficiency.

Whatever the inducing factor(s) are, adult offspring of diabetic and malnourished mothers develop gestational diabetes, and thereby induce a diabetogenic tendency also in their fetuses, and in the consecutive generations.

Lessons from experimental research for the human

The presented data result from experimental work on laboratory models. These animals are bred to form a genetically homogeneous group; the alterations induced in the intra-uterine environment, and the conditions postnatally, are standardized. The effects on the offspring, fetal and adult, are general with minor fluctuations within the experimental groups. The situation in the human is of course much more complicated. The genetic background is heterogeneous, even within a family, and the characteristics of the intrauterine environment are different for each pregnancy, even within the same mother. The adaptation in the fetus and the evolution of the lasting consequences therefore will be heterogeneous. They will not appear in each individual, and not to the same extent in those affected. The results are rather expressed in percentage of incidence of the effect.

However, despite the difficulties in separating genetic and environmental factors, a number of epidemiological studies have been published that clearly point to the lasting influences of the intra-uterine milieu, also in the human.

■ Maternal diabetes

An increased incidence of NIDDM and of gestational diabetes is seen in children of diabetic mothers as compared to those of diabetic fathers [56]. There is a higher incidence of diabetes in descenders from diabetic great-grand mothers via the maternal line than via the paternal line [57]. A significant reduction is found in the incidence of diabetes in children from diabetic mothers, after starting a systematic treatment of diabetic pregnant women [58]. In the Pima Indians, the prevalence of impaired glucose tolerance, of NIDDM and of gestational diabetes, is much higher in children from mothers who had diabetes during that particular pregnancy, than in children from mothers who developed diabetes only after that pregnancy. In the "inheritance" of diabetes in this population, the intra-uterine environment plays a more important role than real genetic heredity [59]. In populations with a normal incidence of diabetes, it has been shown that fetal or neonatal hyperinsulinemia, as seen in diabetic pregnancies, are a strong predictor for the development of impaired glucose tolerance in these children [60]. Also, the difference that we have described between offspring of MD and SD mothers can be recognized. Children from gestationally diabetic mothers develop impaired glucose tolerance, while children from diabetic mothers show early insulin resistance [61]. From these studies it is clear that also in the human, fetal development in a diabetic intra-uterine milieu can induce a diabetogenic tendency in the offspring, without genetic interference.

■ Maternal malnutrition

Also in the human, not only maternal diabetes, but also nutritional factors in the perinatal period can induce a diabetogenic tendency in the offspring. The effect of maternal malnutrition on the health of the children is described in a study on the Dutch hunger winter of 1944 [5]. A previously well-fed population was deprived of food during a 6-month period in the second world war and also pregnant women where thereby forced to severe starvation during a limited period of time. This malnutrition during pregnancy resulted in a higher incidence of impaired glucose tolerance and NIDDM (and cardio-vascular risks) in these children in later life, especially when deprivation occurred during the third trimester. Ample epidemiological studies have documented that low birth weight, particularly thinness at birth, is associated with impaired glucose tolerance, NIDDM [62], hypertension [63] and coronary heart disease [64] in later life. These data are confirmed by several other population studies relating birth weight with adult disease [4, 65–67]. Unfortunately these studies are mostly performed on men, and no data are available on the incidence of gestational diabetes. However, it is likely to be increased as well, since a diabetogenic tendency is clearly transmitted from mother to child. These data point the attention to the importance of maternal nutrition during pregnancy. Temporary or chronic malnutrition of mothers, as it is common in developing countries, can induce impairment of glucose tolerance in the offspring, with gestational diabetes in the pregnant daughters. A vicious cycle of inheritance of gestational diabetes from one generation to another is thereby initiated.

General conclusion

It can be concluded that fetal development in an abnormal intra-uterine milieu indeed can induce lasting consequences for the metabolism of the offspring. Persistent deterioration of the glucose tolerance of the youngsters, especially during pregnancy, can transmit the effect even to further generations. The inducing factors for this transgeneration effect are related to the particular characteristics of the intra-uterine milieu and the resulting body fuels that reach the fetus. Alterations in fetal insulinemia resulting from these adaptations, influence birth weight and explain its correlation with later glucose intolerance. Experimental research in models with altered metabolism during pregnancy should further extend our understanding of the mechanisms involved.

References

[1] Pettitt DJ, Aleck KA, Baird HR, Carraher MJ, Bennett PH, Knowler WC. Congenital susceptibility to NIDDM. Role of intrauterine environment. *Diabetes* 1988; 37: 622-628.

[2] Hales CN. Fetal nutrition and adult diabetes. *Sci Am Sci Med* 1994; 1: 54-63.

[3] Baird J, Phillips DIW. Birth weight and adult disease. In: Dornhorst A, Hadden DR, Eds. Diabetes and pregnancy. An international approach to diagnosis and management. Chichester: John Wiley and Sons, 1996: 377-389.

[4] Lithell HO, Mckeigue PM, Berglund L, Mohsen R, Lithell UB, Leon DA. Relation of size at birth to non-insulin dependent diabetes and insulin concentrations in men aged 50-60 years. *BMJ* 1996; 312: 406-410.

[5] Ravelli ACJ, Van Der Meulen JHP, Michels RPJ, Barker DJP, Hales CN, Bleker OP. Glucose tolerance in adults after prenatal exposure to famine. *The Lancet* 1998; 351: 177.

[6] Fowden AL. The role of insulin in fetal growth. *Early Hum Dev* 1992; 29: 177-181.

[7] Aerts L, Holemans K, Van Assche FA. Maternal diabetes during pregnancy: consequences for the offspring. *Diabetes Metab Rev* 1990; 6:147-167.

[8] Wang C, Hu SM. Developmental regulation in the expression of rat heart glucose transporters. *Biochem Biophys Res Commun* 1991; 177:1095–1100.

[9] Kervran A, Guillaume M, Jost A. The endocrine pancreas of the fetus from diabetic pregnant rat. *Diabetologia* 1978; 15: 387-393.

[10] Sodoyez-Goffaux F, Sodoyez JC, Thiry-Moris YM, De Vos JC. Maturation of liver handling of insulin in the rat fetus. *Diabetes* 1982; 31: 60-69.

[11] De Gasparo M, Milner GR, Norris PD, Milner RD. Effect of glucose and amino acids on foetal rat pancreatic growth and insulin secretion in vitro. *J Endocrinol* 1978; 77: 241-248.

[12] Kervran A, Randon J. Development of insulin release by fetal rat pancreas in vitro: effects of glucose, amino acids, and theophylline. *Diabetes* 1980; 29: 673-678.

[13] Phillips AF, Rosenkrantz TS, Lemons JA, Knox I, Porte PJ, Raye JR. Insulin-induced alterations in amino acid metabolism in the fetal lamb. *J Dev Physiol* 1990; 13: 251-259.

[14] Norberg S, Powell TL, Jansson T. Intrauterine growth restriction is associated with a reduced activity of placental taurine transporters. *Ped Res* 1998; 44: 233-238.

[15] Chen XC, Pan ZL, Liu DS, Han X. Effect of taurine on human fetal neuron cells: proliferation and differentiation. *Adv Exp Med Biol* 1998; 442: 397-403.

[16] Bustamante J, Alonso FJ, Lobo M, Giné E, Tamarit-Rodriguez J, Solis J, Martin Del Rio J. Taurine levels and localization in pancreatic islets. In: Schaffer et al, Eds. Taurine 3. New York: Plenum Press, 1998: 65-69.

[17] Cherif H, Reussens B, Dahri S, Remacle C, Hoet JJ. Stimulatory effects of taurine on insulin secretion by fetal rat islets cultured in vitro. *J Endocrinol* 1996; 151: 501-506.

[18] Plagemann A, Heidrich I, Rohde W, Gotz F, Dorner G. Hyperinsulism during differentiation of the hypothalamus is a diabetogenic and obesity risk factor in rats. *Neuroendocrinol Lett* 1992; 5: 373-378.

[19] Aerts L, Holemans K, Van Assche FA. Impaired insulin response and action in offspring of severely diabetes rats. In: Shafrir E, Eds. Frontiers in diabetes research. Lessons from animal diabetes III. 1990: 561-566.

[20] Ktorza A, Girard J, Kinebanyan MF, Picon L. Hyperglycaemia induced by glucose infusion in the unrestrained pregnant rat during the last three days of gestation: metabolic and hormonal changes in the mother and the fetuses. *Diabetologia* 1981; 21: 569-574.

[21] De Mazencourt P, Carneiro EM, Atroater I, Boschero AC. Prolactin treatment increases Glut2 but not the Gprotein subunit content in the cellmembranes from cultured neonatal rat islets. *FEBS Lett* 1994; 343: 137-140.

[22] Neufeld ND, Corbo L, Kaplan SA. Plasma membrane insulin receptors in fetal rabbit lung. *Pediatr Res* 1981; 15:1058–1062.

[23] Santalucia T, Camps M, Castello A. Developmental regulation of Glut1 and Glut4 glucose transporter expression in rat hearth, skeletal muscle and brown adipose tissue. *Endocrinology* 1992; 130: 837-846.

[24] Philipps AF, Dubin JW, Raye JR. Effect of endogenous insulin release on fetal alanine concentration and uptake. *Am J Obstet Gynecol* 1981; 139: 22-26.

[25] Aerts L, Van Bree R, Feytons V, Rombauts W, Van Assche FA. Plasma amino acids in diabetic pregnant rats and in their fetal and adult offspring. *Biol Neonate* 1989; 56: 31-39.

[26] Mulay S, Philip A, Solomon S. Influence of maternal diabetes on fetal rat development: alteration of

insulin receptors in fetal liver and lung. *J Endocrinol* 1983; 98: 401-410.

[27] Philipps AF, Rosenkrantz TS, Grunnet ML, Connolly ME, Porte PJ, Raye JR. Effects of fetal insulin secretory deficiency on metabolism in fetal lamb. *Diabetes* 1986; 35: 964-972.

[28] Canavan JP, Goldspink DF. Maternal diabetes in rats. II. Effects on fetal growth and protein turnover. *Diabetes* 1988; 37: 1671-1677.

[29] Snoeck A, Remacle C, Reusens B, Hoet JJ. Effect of a low protein diet during pregnancy on the fetal rat endocrine pancreas. *Biol Neonate* 1990; 57: 107-118.

[30] Dahri S, Snoeck A, Reusens-Billen B, Remacle C, Hoet JJ. Islet function in offspring of mothers on low-protein diet during gestation. *Diabetes* 1991; 40(suppl 2): 115-120.

[31] Dahri S, Reusens B, Remacle C, Hoet JJ. Nutritional influences on pancreatic development and potential links with non-insulin-dependent diabetes. *Proc Nutr Soc* 1995; 54: 345-356.

[32] Petrik J, Reusens B, Arany E, Remacle C, Coelho C, Hoet JJ, Hill DJ. A low protein diet alters the balance of islet cell replication and apoptosis in the fetal and neonatal rat and is associated with a reduced pancreatic expression of insulin-like growth factor-II. *Endocrinology* 1999; 140: 4861-4873.

[33] Cherif H, Reusens B, Ahn MT, Hoet JJ, Remacle C. Effects of taurine on the insulin secretion of rat fetal islets from dams fed a low-protein diet. *J Endocrinol* 1998; 159: 341-348.

[34] Holemans K, Verhaeghe J, Dequeker J, Van Assche FA. Insulin sensitivity in adult female offspring of rats subjected to malnutrition during the perinatal period. *J Soc Gynecol Invest* 1996; 3: 71-77.

[35] Garafano A, Czernichow P, Bréant B. Beta-cell mass and proliferation following late fetal and early postnatal malnutrition in the rat. *Diabetologia* 1998; 41: 1114-1120.

[36] Garafano A, Czernikow P, Breant B. In utero undernutrition impairs rat beta cell development. *Diabetologia* 1997; 40: 1231-1234.

[37] Petrik J, Arany E, Mcdonald T, Hill D. Apoptosis in the pancreatic islet cells of the neonatal rat is associated with a reduced expression of insulin-like growth factor II that may act as survival factor. *Endocrinology* 1998; 139: 2994-3004.

[38] Aerts L, Vercruysse L, Van Assche FA. The endocrine pancreas in virgin and pregnant offspring of diabetic pregnant rats. *Diab Res Clin Pract* 1997; 38: 9-19.

[39] Ktorza A, Gauguier D, Bihoreau MT, Berthault MF, Picon L. Adult offspring from mildly hyperglycemic rats show impairment of glucose regulation and insulin secretion which is transmissible to the next generation. In: Shafrir E, Ed. Frontiers in diabetes research. Lessons from animal diabetes. 1990: 555-560.

[40] Oh W, Gelardi NL, Cha CJ. Maternal hyperglycemia in pregnant rats: its effect on growth and carbohydrate metabolism in the offspring. *Metabolism* 1988; 37: 1146-1151.

[41] Susa JB, Boylan JM, Sehgal PK, Schwartz R. Impaired insulin secretion after intravenous glucose in neonatal rhesus monkeys that had been chronically hyperinsulinemic in utero. *Proc Soc Exp Biol Med* 1992; 199: 327-331.

[42] Holemans K, Van Bree R, Verhaeghe J, Aerts L, Van Assche FA. In vivo glucose utilization by individual tissues in virgin and pregnant offspring of severely diabetic rats. *Diabetes* 1993; 42: 530-536.

[43] Ryan EA, Liu D, Bell RC, Finegood DT, Crawford J. Long-term consequences in offspring of diabetes in pregnancy: studies with syngeneic islet-transplanted streptozotocin-diabetic rats. *Endocrinology* 1995; 136: 5587-5592.

[44] Desai M, Crowther NJ, Lucas A, Hales CN. Organ-selective growth in the offspring of protein-restricted mothers. *Br J Nutr* 1996; 76: 591-603.

[45] Sener A, Reussens B, Remacle C, Hoet JJ, Malaisse WJ. Nutrient metabolism in pancreatic islets from protein malnourished rats. *Biochem Mol Med* 1996; 59: 62-67.

[46] Iglesias-Barreira V, Ahn MT, Reusens B, Dahri S, Hoet JJ, Remacle C. Pre-and postnatal low protein diet affect pancreatic islet blood flow and insulin release in adult rats. *Endocrinology* 1996; 137: 3797-3801.

[47] Bennis-Taleb N, Remacle C, Hoet JJ, Reussens B. A low protein isocaloric diet during gestation affects brain development and alters permanently cerebral cortex blood vessels in rat offspring. *J Nutr* 1999; 129: 1613-1619.

[48] Blondeau B, Garafano A, Czernikov P, Bréant B. Age-dependent inability of the endocrine pancreas to adapt to pregnancy: a long-term consequence of perinatal malnutrition in the rat. *Endocrinology* 1999; 140: 4208-4213.

[49] Holemans K, Gerber RT, Meurrens K, De Clercq F, Poston L, Van Assche FA. Maternal food restriction in the second half of pregnancy affects vascular function but not blood pressure of rat female offspring. *Brit J Nutr* 1999; 81: 73-79.

[50] Garafano A, Czernichow P, Bréant B. Effect of ageing on beta-cell mass and function in rats malnourished during the perinatal period. *Diabetologia* 1999; 42: 711-718.

[51] Langley-Evans SC. GDSaJA: Association of disproportionate growth of fetal rats in late gestation with raised systolic blood pressure in later life. *J Reprod Fertil* 1996; 106: 307-312.

[52] Holemans K, Gerber RT, Meurrens K, Declerck F, Poston L, Van Assche FA. Streptozotocin diabetes in the pregnant rat induces cardiovascular dysfunction in adult offspring. *Diabetologia* 1999; 42: 81-89.

[53] Aerts L, Van Assche FA. Ultrastructural evaluation of B-cell recruitment in virgin and pregnant offspring of diabetic mothers. *Diab Res Clin Pract* 1998; 41: 9-14.

[54] Leturque A, Burnol AF, Ferre P, Girard J. Pregnancy-induced insulin resistance in the rat: assessment by glucose clamp technique. *Am J Physiol* 1984; 246: E25-E31.

[55] Holemans K, Aerts L, Van Assche FA. Evidence for an insulin resistance in the adult offspring of pregnant streptozotocin-diabetic rats. *Diabetologia* 1991; 34: 81-85.

[56] Martin AO, Simpson JL, Ober C, Freinkel N. Frequency of diabetes mellitus in mothers of probands with gestational diabetes: possible maternal influence on the predisposition to gestational diabetes. *Am J Obstet Gynecol* 1985; 15:151: 471–475.

[57] Dorner G, Steindel E, Thoelke H. Evidence for decreasing prevalence of diabetes mellitus in childhood apparently produced by prevention of hyperinsulinism in the foetus and newborn. *Exp Clin Endocrinol* 1984; 84: 134-142.

[58] Dorner G, Plagemann A, Reinagel H. Familial diabetes aggregation in type I diabetics: gestational diabetes an apparent risk factor for increased diabetes susceptibility in the offspring. *Exp Clin Endocrinol* 1987; 89: 84-90.

[59] Pettitt DJ. Diabetes in subsequent generations. In: Dornhorst, Hadden, Eds. Diabetes and pregnancy. An international approach to diagnosis and management. Chichester: Wiley, 1996: 367-376.

[60] Silverman BL, Metzger BE, Cho NH, Loeb CA. Impaired glucose tolerance in adolescent offspring of diabetic mothers. Relationship to fetal hyperinsulinemia. *Diabetes Care* 1995; 18: 611-617.

[61] Plagemann A, Harder T, Kohlhoff R, Rohde W, Dorner G. Glucose tolerance and insulin secretion in children of mothers with pregestational IDDM or gestational diabetes. *Diabetologia* 1997; 40: 1094-1100.

[62] Barker DJ, Hales CN, Fall CH, Osmond C, Phipps K, Clark PM. Type 2 (non-insulin-dependent) diabetes mellitus, hypertension and hyperlipidaemia (syndrome X): relation to reduced fetal growth. *Diabetologia* 1993; 36: 62-67.

[63] Barker DJ. Fetal origins of coronary heart disease. *BMJ* 1995; 311: 171–174.

[64] Phillips DI, Barker DJ, Hales CN, Hirst S, Osmond C. Thinness at birth and insulin resistance in adult life. *Diabetologia* 1994; 37: 150–154.

[65] Yajnik CF, Fall CHD, Vaidya U. Fetal growth and glucose and insulin metabolism in four-year old Indian children. *Diabetic Med* 1995; 12: 330-336.

[66] Leon DA, Koupilova I, Lithell HO, Berglund L, Mohsen R, Vagero D, Lithell UB, Mckeigue PM. Failure to realise growth potential in utero and adult obesity in relation to blood pressure in 50 year old Swedish men. *BMJ* 1996; 312: 401-406.

[67] Baird J, Phillips DIW. Birth weight and adult disease. *In:* Diabetes and pregnancy. An international approach to diagnosis and management. Edited by Dornhorst A and Hadden DR. Chichester, John Wiley and Sons. 1996: 377–389.

Test yourself – Questions/Answers

Chapter 1 – Gestational diabetes mellitus: pathophysiology, screening and diagnosis, and management

1. *Gestational diabetes mellitus (GDM) is defined as:*
   a. Any form of carbohydrate intolerance or diabetes occurring during pregnancy
   b. Any form of carbohydrate intolerance or diabetes with onset or first recognition during pregnancy
   c. Any form of carbohydrate intolerance that disappears after pregnancy
   d. Carbohydrate intolerance, but not diabetes, occurring during pregnancy
   e. Any form of carbohydrate intolerance during pregnancy, for which insulin treatment is not required

2. *From a pathophysiological viewpoint, GDM – as compared with normal pregnancies – is characterized by:*
   a. Decreased tissue insulin sensitivity and impaired insulin secretory response
   b. Decreased tissue insulin sensitivity and compensatory insulin secretory response
   c. Normal tissue insulin sensitivity and impaired insulin secretory response
   d. Increased tissue insulin sensitivity and impaired insulin secretory response
   e. Increased tissue insulin sensitivity and compensatory insulin response

3. *The laboratory test with best sensitivity and specificity to screen for GDM is:*
   a. Random plasma glucose within 2 hours of a meal
   b. Random plasma glucose more than 2 hours after a meal
   c. Glycohemoglobin measurement
   d. Glucose challenge test more than 2 hours after a meal
   e. Glucose challenge test in either fasting or fed state

4. *Plasma glucose levels after a GCT shows the following pattern with regard to time since last meal:*
   a. There is no change in plasma glucose with longer interval since last meal
   b. Plasma glucose decreases with longer interval since last meal
   c. Plasma glucose increases with longer interval since last meal
   d. Plasma glucose shows a U-shaped curve with trough values 1-2 hours after last meal
   e. Plasma glucose shows a hyperbolic curve with peak values 1-2 hours after last meal

5. *Pregestational risk factors for GDM do not include one of the following factors:*
   a. Increased bodyweight
   b. Tall stature
   c. Current smoking
   d. Asian ethnicity
   e. PCO syndrome

Answers:
1b; 2a; 3e; 4d; 5b.

Chapter 2 – The inheritance and development of diabetes mellitus

1. *In the absence of classical symptoms, which of the following would confirm the diagnosis of diabetes?*
   a. A single fasting laborator glucose of 12.0 mmol l^{-1}
   b. Two separate office metre readings greater than 13 mmol/l
   c. A laboratory blood glucose reading of 16.6 mmol l^{-1}, 2 hours following a 75 g oral glucose load
   d. Two fasting laboratory blood glucose readings of 7.5 mmol l^{-1} on two consecutive days
   e. A random laboratory glucose of 18.0 mmol l^{-1}

2. *The development of Type 1 diabetes mellitus is **not** associated with:*
   a. Particular haplotypes of the MHC class III gene complex
   b. Particular haplotypes of the MHC class II gene complex
   c. Rubella embryopathy
   d. A short number of repeats of the VNTR in the insulin gene promoter
   e. A low level of insulin expression in the fetal thymus

3. *Islet cell autoantibodies:*
   a. Are always detectable at diagnosis in type 1 diabetes
   b. Are produced by autoreactive T-lymphocytes
   c. May be detected in early childhood
   d. When detected signal the inevitable development of diabetes
   e. Are directed against antigens which show sequence homology to some bacterial antigens

4. *In Type 2 Diabetes:*
   a. There is a requirement for isuelin and patients are prone to ketoacidosis
   b. There is both a failure of insulin secretion and increased insulin resistance
   c. Major genetic causes are well characterised
   d. There is an autoimmune destruction of the pancreatic beta cells
   e. Impaired glucose tolerance always progresses to the development of diabetes

5. *Maturity onset diabetes of the young (MODY):*
   a. Is usually shows an autosomal recessive inheritance pattern
   b. Is inherited through the maternal line
   c. Is frequently associated with sensorineural deafness
   d. Usual onset is before the age of 25 years
   e. Usually shows an X-linked inheritance pattern

Answers:
1d; 2a; 3c; 4b; 5d.

Chapter 3 – Preconceptional care in type I diabetes

1. *An increased incidence of congenital malformations in diabetes and pregnancy is related to:*
    a. Poor metabolic control, early in pregnancy
    b. Hypertension
    c. Menstrual abnormalities
    d. Hypoglycaemia

2. *The most important goal of preconceptional care in diabetes and pregnancy is:*
    a. To prevent sexually transmitted diseases
    b. To obtain normoglycaemia before conception
    c. To avoid vascular complication
    d. To reduce hospital admission

3. *Congenital malformations in diabetes and pregnancy are not related with:*
    a. Duration of diabetes
    b. Severity of diabetes
    c. Vascular complications
    d. Pre-eclampsia

4. *We have not yet realised preconceptional care for every diabetic woman. Indicate strategies to improve the participation of diabetic women in this programme:*
    a. National and international health authorities need to be convinced about the importance of perinatal medicine
    b. Diabetic women should receive information about preconceptional care when receiving diabetic care
    c. Only diabetic women who received preconceptional care will receive financial support during pregnancy and childbirth
    d. Care programmes on diabetes and pregnancy need to be multidisciplinary

5. *Preconceptional care has also an economic benefit and this for the following reasons:*
    a. Reducing perinatal morbidity
    b. Less hospital admission during pregnancy
    c. Preventing diseases in adulthood
    d. A lower insulin regimen during pregnancy

Answers:
1a; 2b; 3d; 4a,b,d; 5a,b,c.

Chapter 4 – Abortion and congenital malfunctions

1. *Which of the following factors is the most important for the risk of congenital malformations in the offspring of a diabetic mother?*
   a. Control of maternal glucose homeostasis during the first trimester
   b. Control of maternal glucose homeostasis during the second trimester
   c. Control of maternal glucose homeostasis during the third trimester
   d. Age of the mother
   e. Size of the fetus

2. *Excess of ROS (Reactive Oxygen Species) is likely to be involved in the pathogenesis of the following conditions associated with diabetic pregnancy;*
   a. Increased fetal movements
   b. Enhanced glucose uptake
   c. Enhanced glycation of proteins
   d. Excessive fetal growth
   e. Pre-eclampsia

3. *Which of these are known teratogens in diabetic pregnancy?*
   a. Diminished arachidonic acid metabolism, increased inositol uptake
   b. Increased glycation of proteins, diminished arachidonic acid uptake
   c. Enhanced ROS formation, diminished inositol uptake
   d. Lowered ROS formation, increased glycation of proteins
   e. Increased arachidonic acid metabolism, diminished inositol uptake

Answers:
1a; 2e; 3c.

Chapter 5 – Medical management of pregestational diabetes

1. *Ultrasound provides information in the 1st trimester*
   a. On viability of the embryo
   b. Accurate estimate of fetal gestational age
   c. Detects congenital malformations

2. *Ulrasound provides information in the 2nd trimester*
   a. Detects structural congenital malformations
   b. Detects chromosome abnormalities
   c. Identifies the macrosomic fetus

3. *Ultrasound provides information in the 3rd trimester*
   a. Can be used to calculate an accurate fetal weight
   b. Identify the disproportionately obese fetus
   c. Give an estimate of fetal lung maturity

4. *The pregestational diabetic mother with background retinopathy is at increased risk of progression of retinopathy*
   a. If glycaemic control is poor periconceptionally and rapidly improves
   b. If anaemic
   c. If pregnancy complicated by hypertension

5. *Hypertension, proteinuria and renal impairment in pregnancy*
   a. Are associated especially with macrosomia
   b. Are associated with increased incidence of PET
   c. Are associated with a premature delivery

6. *The role of home blood glucose monitoring*
   a. Is to gain a detailed profile throughout the day of blood glucose levels
   b. Is to aid in the adjustment and timing of insulin doses
   c. Is to determine the best time for delivery

7. *Neonatal hypoglycaemia (BG < 2.5 mmol/l)*
   a. Neonatal hypoglycaemia is commoner in premature infants
   b. Neonatal hypoglycaemia correlates closely with birth weight
   c. Neonatal hypoglycaemia if not corrected can lead to irreversible brain damage

Answers:
1a,b; 2a; 3b; 4a,c; 5b,c; 6a,b; 7c.

Chapter 6 – Care of the pregnant diabetic woman

1. *The principal foetal anomalies that are related to pre-pregnancy diabetes mellitus are:*
   a. Trisomy 18
   b. Cardiac anomalies
   c. Biliary atresia
   d. Trisomy 21
   e. Renal anomalies

2. *The recommended diet of diabetic women during pregnancy is:*
   a. Hypocaloric and hypolipemic
   b. Balanced normocaloric
   c. Hypocaloric with high-cereal fibre
   d. Hypercaloric with a small quantity of unsaturated fats
   e. A rich fast-absorption carbohydrate diet

3. *The diabetic pregnant women should be surveilled when:*
   a. The fasting glucose levels are 95 mgr/dl or above
   b. One-hour glucose levels after meal is above 140 mg/dl
   c. Two-hour glucose levels after meal is 110 mg/dl or above
   d. There is ketonuria
   e. There is polyhidramnios

4. *The best foetal well-being test for diabetic pregnant women is:*
   a. Manning biophysical score
   b. Doppler ultrasound of uterine arteries
   c. The foetal movement assessment
   d. The oxytocin stress test
   e. The estrogen urine levels study

5. *The delivery should be recommended:*
   a. At 37 week's gestation
   b. Depending on the presence of a macrosomic foetus
   c. At term if there is an appropriate metabolic control and there are no foetal indications
   d. Depending on the foetal breath movements
   e. Depending on obstetrics conditions

Answers:
1b; 2b; 3b; 4a; 5c.

Chapter 7 – Long-term implications of gestational diabetes for the mother

1. *Which of the following physiological changes occur in the mother in normal pregnancy?*
   a. Increased insulin sensitivity
   b. Increased insulin secretion
   c. Pancreatic β cell atrophy
   d. Increased insulin synthesis

2. *Which of the following are independent risk factors for the subsequent development of diabetes in the mother?*
   a. Parity
   b. Gestational diabetes
   c. Obesity
   d. Age

3. *During pregnancy, which of the following maternal findings are predictive of her future development of type 1 but not type 2 diabetes?*
   a. Glutamic acid decarboxylase antibodies
   b. Fasting hyperglycaemia
   c. Islet cell antibodies
   d. Hyperinsulinaemia

4. *Indicate which of the following statements are true:*
   a. Pregnancy is diabetogenic in the long term
   b. The recognition of diabetes for the first time in pregnancy confers an increased risk for subsequent type 2 but not type 1 diabetes
   c. In women with previous gestational diabetes, diet and exercise after the pregnancy may reduce the long-term risk or delay the onset of diabetes
   d. In women with gestational diabetes, there is evidence that oral hypoglycaemic agent therapy during the pregnancy will reduce the long-term risk of diabetes

Answers:
1b,d; 2b,c,d; 3a,c; 4c.

Chapter 8 – Infant of the diabetic mother

1. *Which definition of macrosomia do you consider most appropriate:*
   a. Equal/above 4500 g
   b. Equal/above 4000 g
   c. Equal/above 2 SD of the normal mean value for gestational age and sex

2. *Which infant parameter correlates with achieved degree of maternal blood-glucose control during pregnancy:*
   a. Birthweight
   b. Skinfold thickness
   c. Both(a and b)

3. *What is the current definition of neonatal hypoglycaemia:*
   a. less than 1.7 mmol/1
   b. less than 2.2 mmol/1
   c. less than 2.6 mmol/1

4. *Which pregestational HbA1c level should be aimed at in order to minimize the risk for fetal malformations:*
   a. less than 8 SD above the normal mean value
   b. less than 6 SD above the normal mean value
   c. less than 3 SD above the normal mean value

5. *Which serious long-term morbidity is most likely one in offsprings of type 1 diabetic mothers:*
   a. Obesity
   b. Neurodevelopmental impairment
   c. Type 1 diabetes

Answers:
1c; 2c; 3c; 4c; 5c.

Chapter 9 – Lessons from experimental research: lasting consequences of fetal development in an abnormal intra-uterine milieu

1. *Only one of the following statements concerning* **fetal weight** *is correct:*
   In the experimental model, fetuses of severely diabetic mothers are:
   a. Macrosomic due to fetal hyperglycemia and hyperinsulinemia
   b. Normosomic due to the autonomic glycemic control of the fetus
   c. Microsomic due to deficient nutrient supply from mother to fetus
   d. Microsomic due to a low anabolism as a result of fetal hypoinsulinemia
   e. Microsomic due to deficient food intake by the diabetic mother

2. *Only one of the following statements concerning* **glucose tolerance** *is* <u>not</u> *correct:*
   Deficient insulin response to glucose stimulation in adult offspring of diabetic rat mothers:
   a. Is due to a deficient development of the islets of Langerhans during fetal life
   b. Does not result from a deficient mass of endocrine pancreas
   c. Can be induced by perinatal hyperinsulinemia
   d. Is dependent on the degree of maternal diabetes
   e. Can be associated with low circulating amino acid levels

3. *Only one of the following statements concerning* **gestational diabetes** *is* <u>not</u> *correct:*
   Gestational diabetes in the offspring:
   a. Of diabetic mothers is associated with a deficient islet hyperplasia during pregnancy
   b. Of diabetic mothers is associated with the normal insulin resistance of pregnancy
   c. Is, in its severity, not correlated with the degree of the maternal diabetes
   d. Of diabetic mothers transmits the diabetogenic effect to the male and female offspring
   e. Of severely diabetic mothers produces fetuses with the characteristics of fetuses from mildly diabetic mothers

4. *Only one of the following statements concerning the* **experimental studies** *is* <u>not</u> *correct:*
   a. A normocaloric diet of the pregnant mother can induce an impaired glucose tolerance in the offspring, if the contribution of proteins to the diet is deficient
   b. Even mild gestation of the mother during pregnancy can induce gestational diabetes in the offspring over several generations
   c. Male offspring of diabetic mothers display an impaired glucose tolerance and transmit a diabetogenic tendency to their offspring
   d. Male offspring of diabetic mothers display an impaired glucose tolerance but do not transmit the effect to the next generation
   e. Starvation of the pregnant mother can induce gestational diabetes in her offspring

5. *Only one of the following statements concerning* **human studies** *is* <u>not</u> *correct:*
   Epidemiological studies in the human have shown that:
   a. Gestational diabetes is more frequent in children from diabetic mothers than from diabetic fathers
   b. Systematic treatment of diabetic pregnant women reduces the incidence of diabetes in their offspring

c. Neonatal hyperinsulinemia can be used as a predictor for later glucose intolerance
d. Maternal malnutrition, especially during the first trimester of pregnancy, increases the risk for impaired glucose tolerance in the offspring
e. Low birth weight is associated with impaired glucose tolerance in later life

Answers:
1d; 2a; 3a; 4c; 5d.

Index